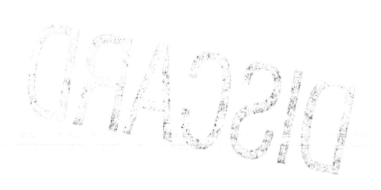

IN HARM'S WAY

A View from the Epicenter of Liberia's Ebola Crisis

by

Nancy D. Sheppard

assisted by Karen J. Gruver

Cover photo by Bethany Fankhauser.

Cover art by Heidi Sheppard Markley

The names of certain individuals mentioned in this book have been changed to protect the privacy of those involved.

IN HARM'S WAY: A VIEW FROM THE EPICENTER OF LIBERIA'S EBOLA CRISIS

To see other books by the author, go to
http://www.sheppards-books.com

Published by Sheppard's Books, USA

Non-fiction missionary story
History of Liberia's Ebola Crisis
ISBN: 978-1-940172-02-6
Sheppard, Nancy, 1960-

Dedicated to
the Ebola fighters in
Liberia, Sierra Leone and Guinea.
I thank God for your dedication
and willingness to risk your lives
to combat this deadly disease.

Contents

Prologue

"Dr. Brantly has tested positive for Ebola!" my son choked out. I gasped in horror and disbelief as I held the phone to my ear, desperately trying to hear my son above the hubbub of the Pennsylvania restaurant's busy Saturday evening crowd. My heart did not want to believe what my ears were hearing.

After John-Mark and I said our goodbyes, I set down the phone, buried my face in the Olive Garden's oversized green napkin and sobbed. When at last I was somewhat composed I looked up at the concerned faces of my husband and my son Jonah. We were having dinner with Timothy and Diane Markley, who were about to become my daughter Heidi's in-laws. None of them could imagine what could have caused such a reaction in me.

"Dr. Brantly has tested positive for Ebola!" I said through sobs. Even as the words came out of my mouth a new and horrible thought came to my mind. "I wonder if this is my fault. Maybe I didn't decontaminate him correctly!"

Timothy Markley jumped in quickly. He reminded me of truths about the sovereignty of God I desperately needed to hear in that moment. These truths would have been impossible to grasp had I not seen God work mightily in so many other desperate situations. Even so, this was unique. The fact was that less than three weeks ago I had worked my last night as a hygienist in the Ebola ward at Liberia's ELWA Hospital—the same ward where Dr. Brantly worked.

After finishing our meal my family and I returned to our hotel, emotionally spent. As I read the first online news of Dr. Brantly's diagnosis, my husband wrote to our prayer supporters, begging them to intercede with God on behalf of this precious young man. Just as he was finishing the email, a Facebook message from a close friend in Liberia left me gasping for breath. "This is not public yet, but Nancy Writebol also tested positive for Ebola this evening. We are all pretty shell-shocked." I melted into a pool of tears.

That night as I sat bathed in the light of the computer screen in a hotel room in Pennsylvania, I could never have imagined the attention Dr. Brantly and Nancy Writebol's positive tests for Ebola would draw to the suffering in West Africa. I had no idea it would catapult the compassionate care of Ebola patients into a spotlight that would lift up the name of Christ around the world. All I knew then was that my friends were most likely going to die very soon and my heart was breaking for them, their families, and for myself.

Chapter 1:
Interesting Times

The well known, albeit apocryphal, Chinese curse, "May you live in interesting times," has been a source of great amusement throughout my life. My "times" have been interesting indeed!

For reasons I have never quite figured out, my college degree in home economics education required three credit hours of zoology for graduation. Unlike its name, which gives the impression the class would be studying zoo animals, we focused on microscopic organisms that could live in the human body—some welcome, but most not so welcome.

If I had paid more attention I might have been a bit more prepared for what lay ahead. Malaria, dysentery, trichinosis, schistosomiasis and a myriad of other exotic illnesses were not considered exotic in my West African life. All that being said, I never, ever, ever—not in my wildest imaginings on my most crazy day—expected to have a working, walking, talking knowledge of Ebola. And yet that is exactly what has happened.

I would say my childhood was very normal, but that would not be quite true. I had Karen, my identical twin sister. We, along with our three brothers, Dan, Paul, and Peter, were raised in Whitewater, Wisconsin, which is a wonderful place to live if you love cold weather. Sadly, I do not.

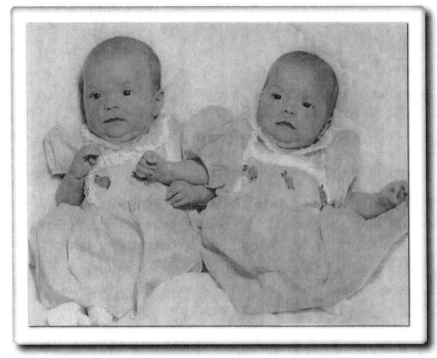

The author Nancy and her assistant Karen (1960)

When we were little, our mom always read Bible stories to us before we went to sleep. When I was five years old she was reading from a book that, for a children's book, had rather graphic pictures. That night's story was about the crucifixion of Christ. The text clearly explained that Jesus was dying for the sins of the world and it was then that I understood for the first time that this included me. My mother asked me if I would like to ask Jesus to be my Savior. I certainly did want that and so, with her help I asked God, in prayer, to forgive my sins and accept me into His family. That same night Karen also accepted Jesus' gift of salvation, making us twins for a second time.

When I was sixteen I met the man who would become my husband. We later attended the same college and got to know each other well. I loved his sense of humor and his apparent lack of fear. He loved that I laughed at his jokes. On a perfectly gorgeous summer day in June of 1980, we were married. A friend sang at our wedding, "Lord, Send Me Anywhere," (by David Livingstone and Faye Lopez) with the pronouns changed from singular to plural. We had no idea God would take our offer so seriously.

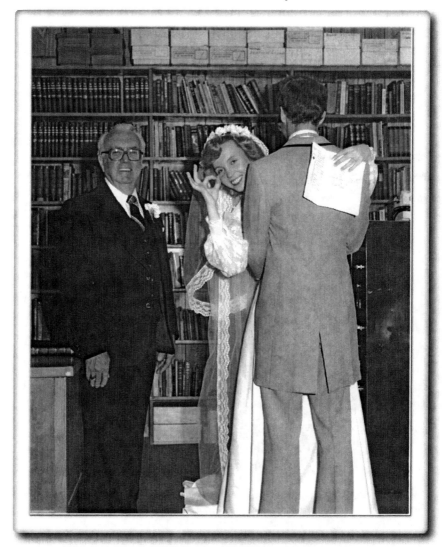

Mark and Nancy with Pastor Reuben Kile on June 21, 1980
(Image - Edward Cunningham)

I finished my last year of college and we settled in Minneapolis, Minnesota, Mark's hometown. In 1982, while attending a mission conference hosted by Valley Baptist, our church in Minneapolis, both Mark and I felt God was asking us to consider foreign mission work. We made an appointment to talk with the main speaker of the conference, Dr. Allen Lewis.

Dr. Lewis was president of Baptist Mid-Missions and was well aware of the opportunities available around the world for missionary volunteers. At our meeting he mentioned an opportunity in Liberia. A group of missionaries wanted to set up a radio station in the interior of the country. After it was on the air, trained Liberian pastors would broadcast Bible lessons in their local languages. Mark, with his degree in broadcast engineering, was immediately intrigued by this project.

In 1986 we moved to Tappita in central Liberia. Three-year-old John-Mark and one-year-old Melodie were with us. I was six months pregnant with Nathan.

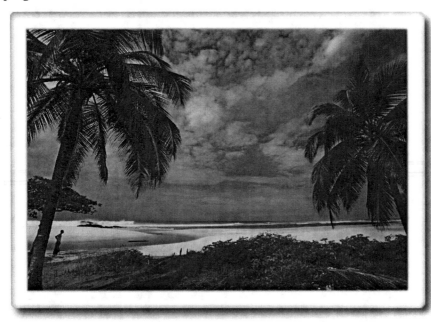

ELWA beach (Image - Bethany Fankhauser)

And I loved it. It thrilled me to be living in West Africa and learning so much about a culture so different from my own in both small and large ways. I loved the beauty of black-brown eyes peering out of smooth, dark skin and the thick crown of braids resting on my friends' heads. I loved that hands were the most important musical instrument and the abandon with which Liberians sang. The elaborate Liberian handshake with its finger snap was fascinating though difficult for a snap-challenged person like me. But most of all I loved the friendliness of the people. Could there possibly be another country in the entire world where every single person I met would greet me back if I smiled and said hello?

The weather was amazing. While some missionaries missed having four seasons, all I cared about was that neither the rainy nor dry season included excessive cold. The easily accessible and gorgeous Atlantic coastline was a treat I could enjoy when we returned from our upcountry home to the capital city of Monrovia for vacations or supply trips.

I loved the rustic beauty of our house and that it sat on a yard in which grew such tropical delights as pineapples, oranges, grapefruit, avocados, cashews and mangoes. I also loved teaching the women and, when given the opportunity, being a bit of an insider to the interesting things happening at the mission's little clinic.

Mark loved the challenge of building a radio station in the middle of the jungle. He also enjoyed teaching in the Bible school, conveniently located on the Tappita mission property, and the simple way of life.

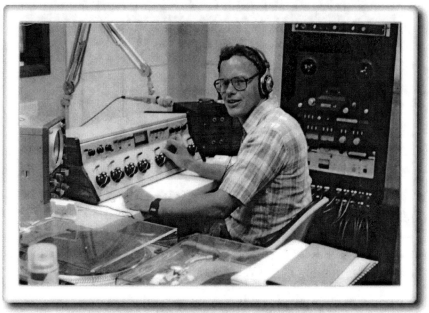

Mark at the controls of the radio station in Tappita

After three wonderful years, we left in June of 1989 for our one-year home assignment. It was during that time the civil war started in Liberia. Because of Liberia's extreme instability, we moved to the

Ivory Coast, Liberia's neighboring country, and began ministering among the war refugees who had fled there. We thought we would be there for no more than six months, the war would end, and we would return to the life we loved so much.

Rather than six months in the Ivory Coast, it was two babies—Heidi and Jared—and twelve years later before we were able to return to Liberia to live.

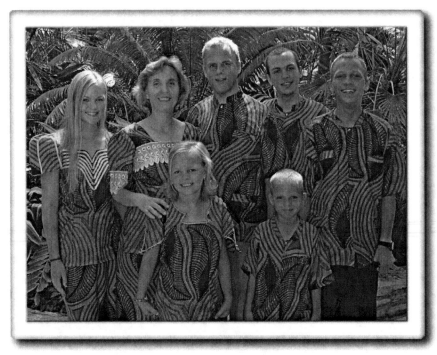

Melodie, Nancy, Heidi, Mark, John-Mark, Jared and Nathan Sheppard (2003)

We settled in Monrovia, Liberia's capital city. I had never been a big-city girl and I did not think I would particularly like living there, but I was wrong. While it was a challenge to work in a country just coming out of a long civil war, there were many things to really love about living in a big city on the ocean.

Being a practical person by nature, I immediately recognized how much easier my life became when I had access to real grocery stores. I felt instantly spoiled by the luxury of being able to cook a wide variety of foods without the weeks of planning ahead that had been necessary while living in the Ivory Coast's interior. The smell of fresh fish filets sizzling in garlic butter was an exotic wonder I never took for granted. The wheelbarrows of used clothing squeaking by the house were the most convenient yard sales ever.

When we traveled into the interior to teach, I enjoyed watching a group of men work together to free a vehicle from a mud hole and their delight at success. I loved the way the Liberian women surged toward me in one fluid motion when I arrived at a conference, singing and dancing their welcome. When it was time for me to leave, they sang a song of God's blessing over me that caused my heart to swell with the joy of knowing them and the privilege of being a part of their lives.

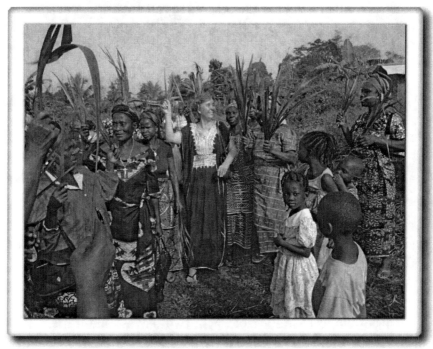

Nancy at a conference in the interior of Liberia

It was fascinating to watch my children grow up in such a place. John-Mark loved the various musical instruments of West Africa, many of which he not only played, but made himself. Melodie had opportunities to care for young children, with whom she was enthralled. My middle child, Nathan, with his effervescent personality, loved meeting strangers at the beach and brought to our dinner table a wide variety of people from around the world. Heidi is artistic to the bone and could capture through the camera lens the beauty of the

Liberian people. Jared, talented in all things electronic, blessed others less gifted, which included me, with his skills.

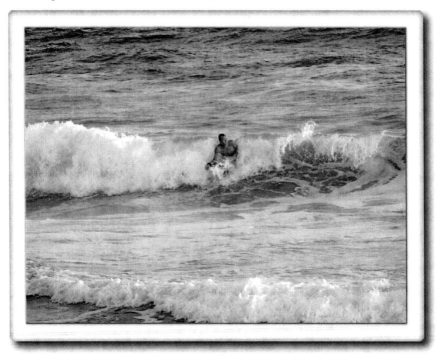

Nathan bodyboarding in Liberia - 2005

I truly enjoyed my ministries in Monrovia, of which there were a wide variety. However, the one I enjoyed the most was hospitality. Friends joked with me that I was always looking for an excuse for a party and I could not deny there was truth to it. Unlike the years in our work among the refugees, in Monrovia I had a big kitchen, a nice-sized dining room, a table with two leaves, and a great set of dishes. I was ready for anything.

Always with an eye out for potential dinner guests, I loved being out and about and meeting new people. The United Nations' contingents were in Liberia with their battalions of men and women. Businessmen and women were arriving, looking for possible opportunity for profit. And of course it was always fun to meet new people with the various mission and non-government organizations (NGOs).

We often socialized with the SIM and Samaritan's Purse missionaries not only because we liked them, which of course we did, but also because they lived on the ELWA campus. ELWA has one of the safest swimming beaches in Monrovia and we tried to take advantage of it at least every two weeks or so. As our children played in the water, we often visited with the missionaries. We loved the ocean and its beauty and we also loved knowing there were like-minded people living near us. After all, we never knew when we would need each other.

Chapter 2:
Portent of Things to Come

Our hearts, already completely intertwined with Liberia and its people, became even more so when God opened a new and completely unexpected door for us in 2005—fostering Liberian children. With the help of our own children, especially Melodie and Heidi, we took in and fostered numerous Liberian babies and toddlers who were later adopted into good homes.

During this process, as we were out and about or when people came from abroad to be united with their children, we were often asked if we planned to adopt a child ourselves. We always replied by saying that if God wanted us to adopt, He would have to make one child stand out.

At the end of 2008, after our one-year home assignment in the States, we flew back to Liberia with Melodie, Heidi and Jared. Melodie, now a young adult, was coming as a short-term missionary. She felt God was leading her back to Liberia to minister in her areas of greatest passion—the discipleship of women and the care of needy children.

After a busy Christmas and New Year conference season in the interior of Liberia we returned to Monrovia, excited to resume fostering. Within weeks we had three little boys sharing our home—two babies and a severely handicapped three year-old. At the end of January an event occurred that would change the course of our lives forever. The Liberian government placed a moratorium on all international adoptions. This sent our world, and that of many others, into a tailspin. I begged God for His mercy on the Liberian children with adoptions in process.

After four months in our home, one of the boys went to live in a well-run special needs orphanage. After sixteen months, because his adoption decree had been signed before the moratorium, another of the boys was allowed to go to his adoptive parents. The last little boy had no such decree and the moratorium remained in place with no end in sight. It gradually dawned on us that this was our "one child," the one we had said God would have to make stand out if He wanted us to adopt.

Two years and nine months after his arrival into our home, Jonah became a Sheppard. Mark and I were awestruck at the cleverness of God. Only He could have arranged a situation so perfectly that we would know beyond doubt this already much-loved child was meant to be *ours*.

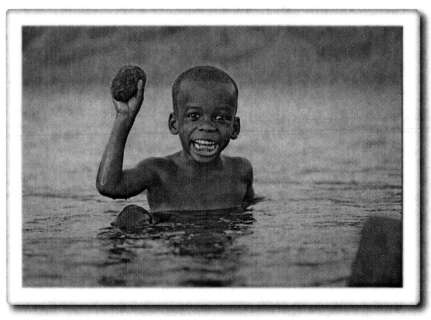

Jonah James Sheppard in 2012 (Image - Heidi Sheppard Markley)

But of course having a young child meant special mommy responsibilities. In August 2013, I was on the ELWA campus engaged in my normal Wednesday afternoon activities—a combination of play date for Jonah, Bible study, errand-running and general socializing—when I met Nancy Writebol for the first time.

David and Nancy, American missionaries new to SIM and Liberia, had arrived the day before. Although they were new to SIM, an evangelical Christian mission agency, this was not the Writebol's first missionary assignment. For fourteen years David and Nancy had worked with needy children in Ecuador and Zambia.

Because I had already invited a neighbor of theirs to dinner, I decided to strike while the iron was hot and invite the Writebols as well. At this dinner we were introduced to each other more thoroughly. As we sat around the table and visited, Nancy and I found we had a lot in common, most notably our passion for missionary work and, of course, our names.

After that first evening at our house, Nancy and I saw each other regularly. Usually it was on the ELWA campus. Wherever there was a job to be done, Nancy was in the middle of it.

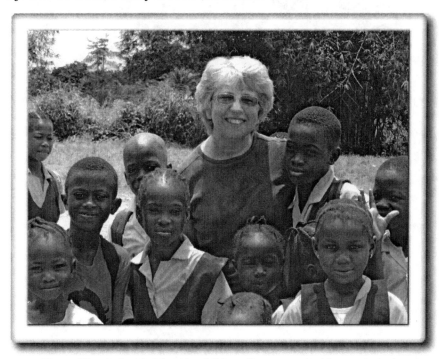

Nancy Writebol with Liberian children (Image used with permission)

Besides our common name, Nancy and I had a common need. Every two months or so I would go to Nancy's little cement-block house where our Dutch friend Aaf would trim our hair while the three of us visited. I always came away looking and feeling better than when I arrived.

In the middle of October another new American family arrived on the ELWA campus—Dr. Kent Brantly, his wife Amber, and their two small children. Kent was working in Liberia under the World Medical Mission's post-residency program, an arm of Samaritan's Purse. Samaritan's Purse was a Christian relief and development agency that had been working in Liberia since the end of their civil war.

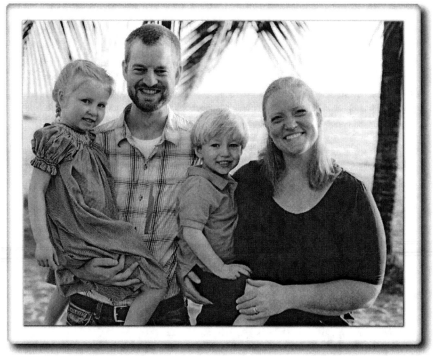

Ruby, Kent, Steven and Amber Brantly at ELWA beach
(Image - Bethany Fankhauser)

Missionary work was not new to the Brantly family either. Kent was only seventeen when he went on his first mission trip to Kenya. Later he traveled to Tanzania, Haiti, Nicaragua, El Salvador and Honduras on other short-term trips. On a trip to Honduras, Kent felt God was calling him to be a missionary doctor. On this same trip he met a lovely nursing student, Amber, who would become his wife.

In November 2013, American SIM missionaries Dr. John Fankhauser and his wife Beth, along with their two teenaged daughters, arrived. After practicing medicine in California, John and Beth felt God leading them to international missionary work. Dr. Fankhauser was immediately busy with hospital duties while Beth and the girls plugged into ministry and social opportunities on the ELWA campus and in the surrounding communities.

While in college God had deeply burdened my oldest son John-Mark to return to Africa to share with the people of West Africa the good news of Jesus Christ. He finished college right around the time Liberia's civil war ended and was able to work with Samaritan's Purse during their early, formative years of post-war ministry.

While a young and single John-Mark was working in Liberia's interior, a mission group from North Carolina visited Liberia. Mark and I knew the team leaders and were invited to join them for dinner one evening. At the end of the meal we were introduced to a lovely young lady from Wisconsin named Sara Dean, who had been regaled through her meal by our daughter Melodie with tales of a young man named John-Mark Sheppard.

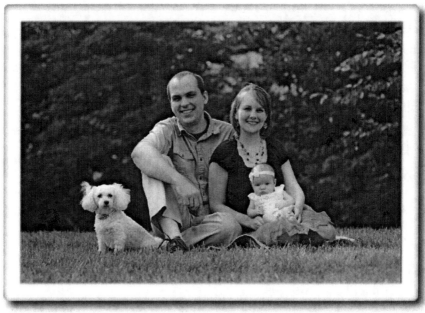

John-Mark, Sara and Audrey Sheppard in 2012 (Image - Melodie Sheppard Kejr)

The next June, after corresponding throughout the year, John-Mark and Sara met face to face. They promptly fell in love and were married the next year. After a few years in the States, they joined SIM and in 2012 returned to Liberia as a couple. With them was my granddaughter Audrey. Sara was pregnant with baby number two. After spending several weeks in Monrovia, they moved to Voinjama in northwestern Liberia. They returned to Monrovia every few months to replenish their supplies. We loved it when they stayed at our home during those trips.

In March 2014, John-Mark and Sara's visit to Monrovia coincided with the missionary picnic—a bi-annual event where the missionary community gathered to eat, share news and fellowship. It was at this wonderful meal, in its idyllic setting by the gorgeous Atlantic shoreline, that I heard the missionary doctors first mention that Ebola had reared its ugly head in neighboring Guinea.

Soon others missionaries were talking about it as well. Of course we had all heard of Ebola. Like other exotic diseases, Ebola lurks just below the consciousness as something remotely possible but ever so unlikely.

Ebola Hemorrhagic Fever (EHF), also known as Ebola Virus Disease (EVD) or simply Ebola, was first identified in 1976. A forty-four year-old man who lived near the Ebola River in Zaire (present-day Democratic Republic of Congo) had the first known case. Ebola's early symptoms include fever, sore throat, muscle pain, headache and extreme weakness. Vomiting, diarrhea and a rash soon follow.

The body's immune system identifies attackers using dendritic cells, which also direct other immune system cells to attack the invaders. However, according to virologists, when Ebola enters the body, it begins by invading the dendritic cells, turning them off. Without the direction provided by the dendritic cells, the immune system seems to know there is an invader, but does not know what it is or what to do about it. The Ebola virus then is free to replicate in the lymphoid tissue and spread throughout the body.[1]

As the disease progresses, the immune system senses the body is in serious trouble, and floods the body with all of the anti-virus weapons in its arsenal. However, without the dendritic cells to control it, the immune system produces what researchers call a "cytokine storm" which attacks every organ in the body, creating holes in the blood vessels. This causes internal bleeding or, in doctor speak,

---

[1] http://www.medicaldaily.com/ebola-explained-what-happens-when-one-worlds-deadliest-viruses-invades-your-immune-system-297130

hemorrhaging. In some cases blood may even come from the eye-balls, ears, mouth and rectum, making a gruesome disease even more grisly. This also is when the body is most infectious since every drop of bodily fluid which leaks from the victim now contains millions of Ebola viruses which are ready to infect someone else.[2] The patients often die either from multiple organ failure or the shock caused by dehydration—many times within days.

It was no simple thing for epidemiologists to figure out how Ebola Hemorrhagic Fever (EHF) got into the population in the first place. Experts now believe fruit bats were the initial carriers. These nocturnal creatures are extremely common in West Africa with sometimes hundreds roosting in a single fruit tree.

When we lived in Tappita during our first three years in Liberia, it was common for a bat to get a piece of fruit from one of the many mango trees around our house and carry it off. When it proved too heavy, the mango would drop with a loud bang on our corrugated roof, waking us up with a start. When we found out the Bible school students enjoyed eating bat meat, at times Mark used his pellet gun to shoot the ones hanging in the trees on the mission property.

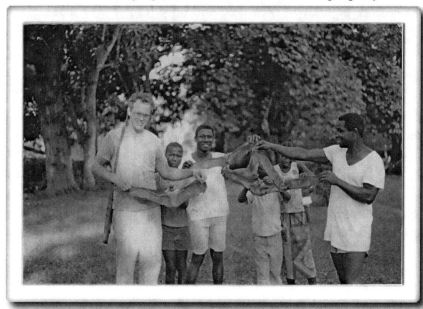

Mark bat hunting with Liberian friends in Tappita, Liberia (1989)

---

[2] http://www.uncommonwisdomdaily.com/ebola-what-you-need-to-know-19064

Experts believe Ebola is passed to humans by contact with the bat's blood or saliva. From there it is spread from human to human. It does not seem necessary for the first human to have touched an actual bat. A piece of fruit dropped by an infected bat could be eaten off the jungle floor by another animal that would then host the virus. If someone butchers that animal, he risks exposure. Some researchers also believe that people might become infected by eating fruit or other uncooked foods contaminated by the droppings of infected bats.

When news of the first confirmed cases of Ebola in Liberia was heard, a collective shudder went through the community of foreigners. A meeting was called for all American citizens. On April 10th Mark, John-Mark, Sara and I made our way to the new U.S. Embassy compound in Mamba Point.

Parking was tight and the seating area full. Among others, Ambassador Deborah Malac herself spoke. She cautioned people to not overreact and flee the country. According to the Center for Disease Control (CDC) and the World Health Organization (WHO), anyone who was walking around doing his daily business could not infect the healthy population. People could only transfer the disease once they were seriously ill.

A handout gave the pertinent facts: The suspected reservoir for Ebola is fruit bats. Transmission to humans is thought to come from infected bats or from primates that have been infected by the bats. Undercooked meat can transfer the virus to humans. Most often human transmission is exclusively among caregivers to the very ill. The virus is easily killed by contact with soap, bleach, sunlight or drying. The virus incubates in humans for two to twenty-one days. The viral load shows itself first in the blood and then later in vomit, feces, urine, semen, tears and sweat. Ebola cannot be contracted through handling of money, buying bread or swimming in a pool. We were told there was no reason to stop normal activities. No flights should be stopped. No borders should be closed. There should be no restriction on travel. There would be no need to close any businesses or schools. We could protect ourselves by not touching anyone who was obviously sick.

We found it all very reassuring and left the embassy in good spirits. It was nearing dusk and thousands upon thousands of fruit bats that live in the gigantic trees near the edge of the embassy property were floating high in the sky like a cloud of huge gnats. The irony was lost on no one.

Embassy meetings notwithstanding, within hours most mission agencies represented in Liberia were discussing their exit strategies. Within a few days SIM and Samaritan's Purse families with young children returned to their home countries.

Our son John-Mark and his family were allowed to stay in Liberia as long as they remained in Monrovia with us rather than returning to Lofa County where the cases of Ebola had been confirmed. Since we did not live near any healthcare center that could bring the disease to our doorstep, we felt the two of our six children who remained in the home would be safe.

I wanted to help in the fight against Ebola. After all, if people like me did not help, who would? I called up Dr. Debbie Eisenhut, an American SIM missionary friend and a surgeon at the ELWA Hospital, to ask how to proceed. She referred me to Keren Massey, the Canadian woman heading up Samaritan's Purse's Ebola response team.

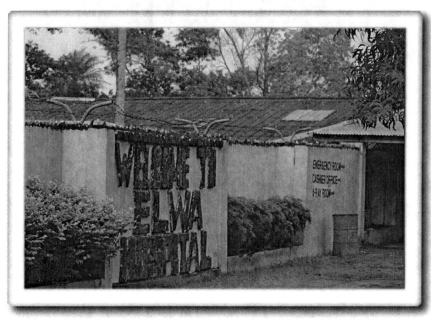

ELWA Hospital entrance (Image - Bethany Fankhauser)

I drove to Samaritan's Purse's headquarters on the ELWA campus. It was familiar territory. I'd known SP's director Kendall Kauffeldt and his wife Bev since their arrival in Liberia not long after the civil war ended. John-Mark had enjoyed their friendship during his time as a Samaritan's Purse employee and our family appreciated their deep and ongoing concern for Liberia and her people.

A receptionist directed me to Keren's office. After getting to know each other a bit, I expressed my interest in volunteering to help in whatever way I could with the present Ebola problem. Knowing our connections with churches and their pastors in Liberia's interior, Keren wondered if I would consider traveling to Nimba County to teach Ebola prevention strategies. I knew that would not work. We had only one vehicle and it was needed in Monrovia. Keren suggested I talk with Nancy Writebol, who was helping to put together the Ebola ward on ELWA's campus.

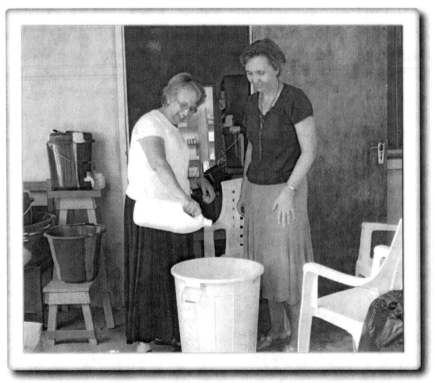

Nancy Writebol training Nancy Sheppard (Image - Dr. Debbie Eisenhut)

At that point I, the queen of volunteering, had not given much thought to how few volunteers there would be for work in an Ebola ward. When I called Nancy, I was pleasantly surprised and somewhat flattered by how genuinely thrilled she was to hear from me. She asked me to meet her at the hospital's chapel right away. Once there, I explained what I was willing to do and Nancy immediately suggested I, like her, be trained to help suit up the doctors and nurses going into the ward and decontaminate them when they came out. That sounded like a good job for me. I could not see any downside to this plan.

Chapter 3:
The Embers Smolder

On December 6, 2013, West Africa's Ebola "Patient Zero," a two year-old boy named Emile, died in the village of Meliandou in southeastern Guinea.[1]

A week later his mother was dead, followed by his three year-old sister and grandmother. Two mourners who attended the grandmother's funeral took the virus home to their village. A health worker carried it to still another village, where he died, as did his doctor. They both infected relatives from other towns.

All of the dead had exhibited similar symptoms—fever, vomiting and diarrhea. But fever, vomiting and diarrhea are common symptoms for a host of other ailments in West Africa. Doctors in Guinea thought it was Cholera. By the time Ebola was identified in March, dozens of people had died in eight Guinean communities.[2]

A traditional healer living in the isolated village of Sokoma, Sierra Leone, claimed to have powers to cure Ebola. People from Guinea crossed the border to take advantage of her skills.[3] Her death from Ebola was followed by a traditional funeral, which involves touching, even kissing, the corpse. Unknowingly, people carried the virus back to their homes. Soon they got sick and died and were honored with traditional funerals as well.

By the end of March, Ebola had begun its grisly march into Libe-

---

[1] http://nypost.com/2014/10/28/ebola-outbreaks-patient-zero-was-a-2-year-old-from-guinea/

[2] http://www.nytimes.com/2014/08/10/world/africa/tracing-ebolas-breakout-to-an-african-2-year-old.html, accessed Oct. 2, 2014.

[3] http://www.timesliv੭.co.za/africa/2014/08/20/sierra-leone-s-365-ebola-deaths-traced-back-to-traditional-healer

ria. Two Liberians who had visited Guinea were struck down with the disease. A week later there were seven, then twenty and then more. Doctors Without Borders (commonly called MSF for its French name Médecins Sans Frontières[4]) began work on an isolation unit in Foya, a town in Lofa County near where John-Mark and Sara lived.

No one wanted Ebola to come to Monrovia, but there was no denying it was a real possibility. Despite their demanding schedules, Dr. Jerry Brown, ELWA Hospital's administrator, along with Dr. Debbie, Dr. Brantly and Dr. Fankhauser, set to work. They felt it vital that, should Ebola ever reach Monrovia, infected people go to an Ebola ward rather than stay in their communities and risk contaminating others. All care would be free of charge.

Every room of the hospital was already being used to the fullest. Fortunately, there was a cement block, corrugated-roofed chapel that the staff used each morning for devotions. It was about the size of a volleyball court inside with full-sized porches running its length on both sides and it was separated from the rest of the complex by a patch of lawn.

The chapel would have to do the job. A plan was drawn up and missionary David Writebol, along with his grounds crew, transformed the chapel into a five-bed ward. Electricity was installed. Beds and other supplies were brought to the site and put in place. Water was brought through a garden hose.

Training was important. Dr. Debbie provided specialized teaching sessions for the nurses. A team of doctors with Doctors Without Borders (MSF) came from Europe to train healthcare workers and volunteers such as Nancy Writebol and me.

Once the ward was set up and the staff trained, there was almost an eerie quiet in Monrovia. No patients came to the ELWA Ebola ward. No patients were admitted to John F. Kennedy Hospital's Ebola ward. A story floated around the city of a sick woman who had taken care of her sister who died of Ebola. There was a rumor that she had stayed overnight in Chicken Soup Factory, a suburb of

---

[4] http://www.msf.org/

Monrovia. Later we heard that the driver of the motorcycle taxi who took her to a hospital had died. We had no way of verifying any of the rumors.

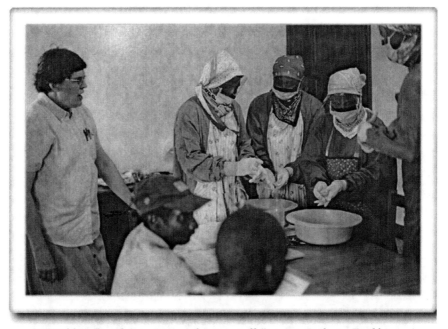

Dr. Debbie Eisenhut training Liberian staff (Image - Bethany Fankhauser)

All we knew for sure was that the expected wave of Ebola patients at ELWA had not materialized. After six weeks in our home, John-Mark and Sara returned to Voinjama. My missionary friends and their young children returned from their evacuation trips, happy to have spent time with family and friends but even happier to be back in their adopted homeland. For most people in Monrovia the Ebola scare was yesterday's news.

Not long after John-Mark and Sara returned to Voinjama, their one year-old son Noah developed an abscess on his arm. It kept getting bigger and redder and his parents were very concerned. They took him to Tellewonyan Hospital, located within two miles of their home, where the abscess was lanced. They were told by the hospital staff to return two days later for the wound to be cleaned and dressed.

The next day Sara called Dr. Debbie in Monrovia to give an update on Noah's infection. Dr. Debbie informed Sara that Tellewonyan Hospital had just received its first Ebola patient. She cautioned them to stay away from the hospital and instructed Sara on how to care for the wound at home. The risk was just too great.

Around that same time a woman infected with Ebola traveled from Sierra Leone to Monrovia, where she stayed with a family in a crowded section of the city called New Kru Town. She got sick and was soon dead. Shortly thereafter a member of the household got sick and visited Monrovia's Redemption Hospital for treatment. The nurse who treated that patient became sick and died.

Around noon on June 12th I received a call from Nancy Writebol. Rather than her normal, perky-sounding voice, I heard only exhaustion. A patient was in the Ebola ward and Nancy had been working since yesterday afternoon. Could I come?

I rearranged my schedule and prepared what I needed to take with me to work through the night. When Mark and I left at two-thirty for ELWA Hospital, I felt a strange mixture of trepidation and excitement. I had never done anything like this before.

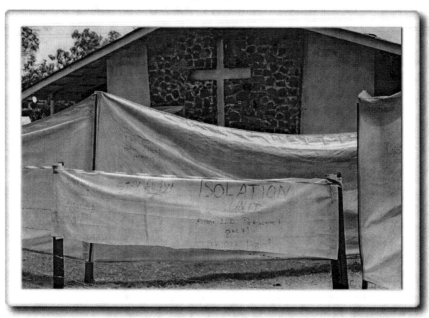

ELWA Hospital's Ebola ward entrance (Image - Bethany Fankhauser)

After being dropped off in front of ELWA's small pharmacy building, I walked the short distance to the Ebola ward, passing through the dozen or so patients waiting to be seen by the doctor. I was on familiar turf. Between my family and the many babies we had fostered, we had taken advantage of ELWA Hospital's services countless times through the years.

I walked past a security guard who sat at a desk and toward the large white plastic tarp stretched on wooden poles to provide privacy for the Ebola ward. Bold, hand-written letters stated, "Stay Away! Isolation unit. Authorized personnel only."

Dr. Debbie and Nancy Writebol stood on the porch, both looking exhausted. After greetings, they filled me in on what was happening. The day before two patients had arrived together—a young lady named Juliet and her uncle. Their symptoms were consistent with Ebola. The uncle had passed away in the two hours it had taken to arrange for admittance.

I walked to the threshold of the door that stood open to the chapel's interior. Lying in a metal hospital bed approximately fifteen feet from me was an extremely sick-looking young lady in a blue hospital gown. While I knew that with time I would learn all the necessary procedures and protocols, in that moment, as I looked at our first Ebola patient, I felt the weight of my decision to volunteer.

I turned back to Dr. Debbie and Nancy. Thankfully they realized I needed more training before being left on my own. Nancy showed me the layout of the building and where all of the supplies were kept. She pointed out that opposite the front porch and under the overhang of the hospital building was a large shelving unit made of cement blocks and wooden planks. These shelves held IV fluids and tubing, body bags, cleaning supplies, towels, gowns and the other items needed in bulk.

At the front end of the chapel near the entrance to the ward was a large walk-in closet, which was used both for storage and as a changing room. On the floor in the closet stood about two dozen pairs of rubber boots and the same number of plastic Crock looka-likes. The boots would be worn into the ward and the other shoes put on when the boots were removed upon exiting. Also in the closet were stacks of folded scrubs, latex gloves, facemasks, medicines and paper plates.

On the porch near the entrance to the ward was a large bookshelf. Folded Tyvek® suits were on the top shelf, arranged by size. These adult-sized "footie pajamas" are disposable garments designed to protect medical workers from contamination. The lower shelves held latex gloves, facemasks, goggles, bed sheets and various medicines.

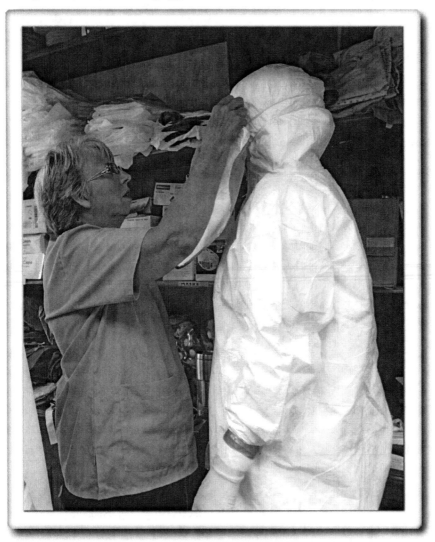

Nancy Writebol preparing a nurse to go into the Ebola ward
(Image - Bethany Fankhauser)

When it was time for Juliet, our patient, to receive her care, Nancy and I worked together to suit up Dr. Debbie and Beatrice, the Liberian nurse assigned to the ward. A Tyvek® suit was put on over scrubs and a pair of knee-high rubber boots. Once the suit was on and zipped up the front, a pair of surgical gloves was taken out of its package and duct taped, with a small end tucked under to create a tab for future removal, under the elasticized wristband of the Tyvek® suit. Another pair of gloves was put over the first pair, this one duct taped on top of the Tyvek® suit. A large plastic apron was next. It was pulled tightly to the neck by the plastic buckle on the right side. Over the hood of the suit was placed a surgical facemask and goggles. To cover any exposed skin around the face, "beards" were cut out of Tyvek® material and duct taped to the sides of the hood.

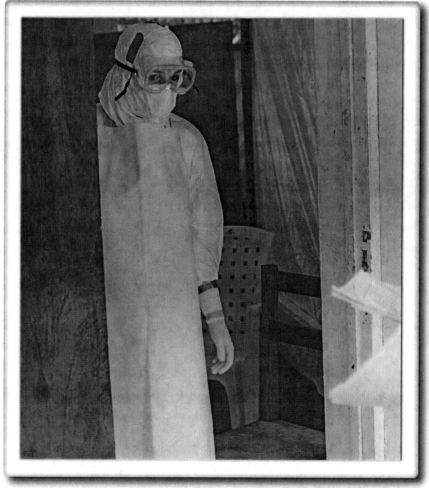

Samaritan's Purse Nurse inside of Ebola ward (Image - Bethany Fankhauser)

As Dr. Debbie and Beatrice were suiting up, a process that took close to half and hour, they discussed what they would do inside the ward and the needed items were gathered. Once they stepped over the threshold, they could not come back until they were completely finished with Juliet's care and had been thoroughly decontaminated.

While Dr. Debbie and Beatrice took care of Juliet in the ward, Nancy explained other responsibilities that were mine. If a doctor or nurse needed something while in the ward, he or she would let me know by calling for me. If the needed item were on the shelves, I would grab it. If it were in the pharmacy, I would go get it. The needed item would then be dropped into a dishpan immediately inside the ward, taking care to touch nothing. If they needed more bleach water, I would carry it to them in a bucket from my trash can-size supply near the disinfecting area. Rather than setting it down, I would pour the water into one of the buckets kept immediately inside the ward on the other side of the all-important threshold.

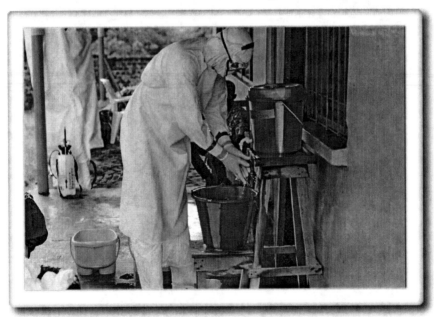

Hand-washing station in decontamination zone of the Ebola ward
(Image - Bethany Fankhauser)

After Dr. Debbie and Beatrice were done in the ward, it was time for me to help them with the decontamination process. The decontamination area was on the porch at the far side of the chapel. I felt nervous because the procedure was both complicated and vitally important. There was no room for error.

Beatrice went first. One foot at a time she stepped into the chlorinated water that was in a rectangular bucket on the ground. Next, gloved hands were washed in chlorinated water under the spigotted bucket that had been placed on a small stand against the wall. After washing hands, carefully pushing the water between each finger, Beatrice cupped her hands and poured water over the top of the spigot to clean off any virus.

The duct tape was then peeled away from the top pair of gloves, which were removed and thrown into a waiting, lined trashcan. Holding arms out in spread-eagle fashion, Beatrice stepped up to to the wooden bar that had been placed as a dividing point between the unsafe and the safe area. With me on one side of the bar and she on the other, I pumped the plunger on the sprayer—the kind found in garden centers to spray for bugs. Once I had water pressure I used the wand to spray her from fingertip to fingertip, across the front of the suit, down the legs and then the same thing on the back side of the suit.

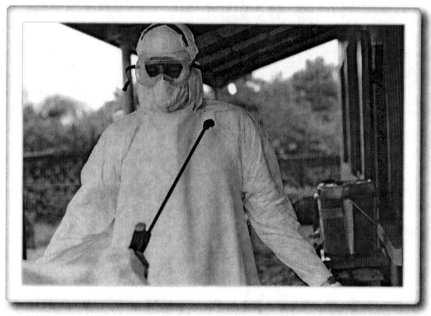

Doctor John Fankhauser being decontaminated as he leaves the Ebola ward
(Image - Bethany Fankhauser)

The apron was then unbuckled, pulled off, and carefully swished by Beatrice in a strategically-placed trashcan of chlorinated water before it was pushed down into yet another trashcan filled with chlorinated water to soak for half an hour. Gloved hands were washed again. The same spray process across the front and then the back of the suit was repeated. Then the goggles were carefully pulled from her eyes, lifted up over the head and then dropped into a waiting bucket of chlorinated water. Gloved hands were washed yet again. The facemask was then removed and hands washed.

The zipper on the front of the Tyvek® suit was carefully pulled down and Beatrice washed her hands again before the duct tape was removed from the inside pair of surgical gloves. Before the gloves were removed, using care her hands did not touch it, the suit was shrugged off her shoulders, down to the ground and pulled over her boots while deliberately trying to turn it inside out. Beatrice, dripping sweat and noticeably relieved to be out of the hot suit, had been instructed to touch only the inside of the Tyvek® suit as she carefully balled it up and placed it in the garbage can. Gloved hands were washed yet again with chlorinated water and the remaining pair of surgical gloves removed.

Pumping up my sprayer again, I sprayed the front and back of both of Beatrice's boots. Then I sprayed the bottom of one boot, which was not set down again, but rather lifted and placed on my side of the line. As Beatrice struggled to stay balanced, I sprayed the second boot bottom and it too was placed on my side of the line. Beatrice then stepped into another footbath and, after that, using a large specially-made wooden shoehorn, the boots were removed—without hands—and placed in yet another trashcan filled with bleach water to soak. Lastly, another hand washing was done, first with bleach water and then fresh. The whole process was repeated with Dr. Debbie.

I also needed a crash course on preparing the chlorinated water, of which we used a lot. The plastic trashcans as well as the hand washing station buckets and cleaning buckets needed refilling and refreshing regularly. Nancy showed me the line on the large trash cans to which the water should be filled. Then a one-gallon jug of bleach was poured in. She was well acquainted with this process as every day since the ward had been made ready, Nancy had changed the bleach water in anticipation of the first Ebola patient.

After I was shown these procedures, I felt fairly confident that I could handle things on my own. Dr. Debbie and Nancy left for their homes to get some much needed sleep.

After resting a few hours, Dr. Debbie returned for the night. While I had always admired her, that night as I visited with her on the porch during down times, I found my esteem for her growing. I already knew she had been a driving force behind the renovations, so determined was she that Ebola patients arriving in Monrovia have a place ready to receive them. Now I was seeing both the eagerness she displayed to teach the Liberian nurses the protocols necessary for keeping themselves safe and the compassion with which she cared for Juliet.

The next morning, when my shift was over, Mark arrived to pick me up. He had with him a thermos of hot coffee and a package of cookies. In the car, as we drove through the busy morning traffic towards home, I tried to explain to Mark what my night was like. There were so many jumbled thoughts in my head that it was hard to articulate them. I felt like I was being allowed into someone else's world. A world I had never, in my wildest imagination, thought I would be a part of.

The next night I worked with Dr. Brantly. I had met him on several occasions, but it was his wife Amber I knew as a friend. Kent was humble, fun and polite as we worked together to help Lydia and David, the two Liberian nurses assigned to the ward, get into their personal protection equipment (PPEs). His ready smile and sweet words assured the nervous nurses that we were going to do our best to keep everyone safe.

After everyone but me was suited up to go into the ward, we carefully looked for any exposed skin. I felt very responsible for these people and sensed the responsibility they felt for each other as well. Once content everyone was properly covered, we gathered in a circle by the threshold going into the ward and joined hands. Dr. Brantly asked me to pray. I prayed for Juliet. I prayed for the team going in to care for her. I prayed for Liberia.

As the team lumbered awkwardly into the ward in their matching white suits, I moved from the doorway about six feet over to the screen block window and peered in. I watched the team move toward Juliet's bed. While the nurses stood to the side of the bed and waited, Dr. Brantly, distinctively tall and thin, walked to the head of the bed and placed his hand gently on Juliet's forehead. His eyes under the mask met hers. I heard him speak. While I could not understand the words, I could hear his soothing tone.

While I watched, tears threatened to overflow my eyes. What am I seeing here? I asked myself. It was invisible to all but me. This dying woman was perhaps the most untouchable person in the world and yet Dr. Brantly was touching her. And he was not just touching her physically, but emotionally and spiritually as well. Who was I that I should be granted the privilege of witnessing this? It was somehow both utterly tragic and supremely glorious.

Chapter 4:
It's Complicated

Our routine was established. Nancy Writebol worked in the daytime and I worked through the night. My main problem was the drive to and from the hospital. The rainy season was upon us and water often flowed over my car's windshield and onto the river-like road as I inched my way through Monrovia's heavy traffic. It often took more than half an hour to travel the eight mile distance.

"You know they're calling us the bleach babes," Nancy Writebol said one night as I stepped onto the chapel's porch. I laughed out loud. It was crazy, but it fit. Our job was to get bleach where it needed to go and the "babes" label was ridiculous enough to be truly funny.

Although we had known each other before, Nancy and I were getting closer. We shared the same responsibility and understood each other's fears. Both of us struggled from time to time with the massive responsibility of what we were doing. The people we were helping to suit up and decontaminate were people we knew and cared about deeply. We were not particularly worried about ourselves since over our scrubs we wore surgical aprons, latex gloves, a facemask and goggles. We were much more concerned that a mistake on our part could cause the deaths of our friends.

The routines became familiar. I helped the doctors and nurses suit up before entering the ward. I decontaminated them when they left the ward. I prepared the garbage cans of bleach water. I went to the pharmacy for drugs. I straightened up and swept the porch. I put the bleached plastic aprons on the line to dry. I hung the bleached rubber boots on the sticks in the yard. But even as the routines became familiar, being in the ward and a part of the team never became old.

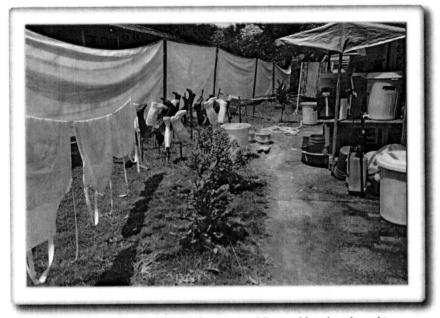

*Drying area (left), final footbath area (middle) and last hand-washing
station (right) in the Ebola ward (Image - Bethany Fankhauser)*

Despite everyone's efforts to save her, Juliet died after just a few
days in the ward. It was very sobering. Following her death, there
were two nights with no Ebola patients. Then fourteen year-old Gartee arrived. He came from the area known as Twelve Houses in Pay-
nesville, where he lived with his uncle and attended an Islamic
school. It was disconcerting to hear that Ebola was in that neighborhood. It later came to light that his family lived in New Kru Town
near the Duala market. He had a friend with whom he played soccer
who had recently died. The friend's housekeeper had come to work
sick. When Gartee started feeling sick, his family recognized it as
potentially Ebola.

Happily for him, perhaps because it was caught so early, Gartee
never got desperately sick. In fact, he was well enough that often he
felt bored in the Ebola ward. Dr. Brantly brought him a soccer ball
and even kicked it around the yard with him, Kent all decked out in
his PPE. When not in use, the ball rested near Gartee's head. Dr.
Brantly also brought him wildlife magazines and David Neff's book,
Stories I Heard in Africa, which my friend Eric Buller read to him in

38

the daytime—Eric on one side and Gartee on the other side of the all-important threshold.

Solomon came soon after. He sold clothing in the Duala market for a living. He did not appear deathly sick at first and even talked briefly on the cell phone he had brought with him. However, after a full day in the ward when the phone rang he did not respond. After only a few days he died.

Hawa and Rose arrived next. They were the mother and young adult sister of a Monrovia nurse who had treated an Ebola patient and died not long after. The two women were placed at the far end of the ward with their beds foot to foot. While they could see each other and talk to each other if they wanted to, they seldom did. Both seemed locked in their own worlds of grief, pain and misery. Soon Rose died. There was no keeping Rose's death from her mother. Too weak to speak, she gestured with her hand hopelessness and despair. Within a week, she too was dead.

A woman came from another Monrovia suburb, Jacobstown. She arrived in the back seat of a taxi sandwiched between two relatives. Like Solomon, she also sold in the Duala market. She was so sick that she passed away before even being removed from the vehicle.

Once the death was confirmed, the bereaved family was preparing to leave, taking the dead woman's body with them for burial. Dr. Brantly, understanding the danger in which they were placing themselves, asked them to reconsider. They were hesitant to comply, so Dr. Brantly got down on his knees and begged them to leave the body with him. Thankfully, in the end they agreed to his request.

A two-year-old girl was brought to ELWA Hospital for treatment. When asked about possible contact with Ebola, the mother was not forthcoming. Because her symptoms seemed suspicious, the little girl was admitted to the Ebola ward. The mother panicked, crying out that if the neighbors found out her child was in the Ebola ward she would not be allowed back into the community. She fled in terror.

The girl was deathly sick and so anemic that some of the staff feared she would die in the night. As I watched from my window, a doctor and three nurses, dressed in their PPEs, hovered over her, discussing her case. She was treated for several obvious symptoms and began to show improvement almost immediately. Her test for Ebola was negative and the little girl was moved to the pediatric ward. Thankfully her mother was found and, after several days of hospital care, the child was able to return to her home.

By this time I realized that every single thing about Ebola in Liberia was complicated and these complications were exacerbating the spread of the virus. This little girl showcased one of the bigger problems. Separating the Ebola cases from the other illnesses presenting themselves in the emergency room was complicated because Ebola had several symptoms similar to other common illnesses. While waiting for test results, the staff had to be very careful. Everything about their care of the undiagnosed patients had to be kept completely separate from the care of those with confirmed cases of Ebola. If a test proved negative, the fortunate patient went through a careful process to exit the ward. The same careful process was used for a patient who survived Ebola.

Blood testing was complicated. To determine if someone had Ebola, blood cultures were sent to the old lab at the Liberian Institute for Biomedical Research. Today it is remembered primarily because of nearby Monkey Island, the "retirement home" for former lab chimps and their offspring. Often we had to wait for a day or two to receive back the results. All blood draws required a health professional to suit up. If the person were alive, blood was drawn from an arm. If the person were dead, blood was drawn by jabbing a needle into the heart of the corpse and extracting it. The testing itself was not straightforward. A person who was just starting to show symptoms could test negative but then test positive a few days later as the viral load increased throughout his body.

The Liberian culture itself presented complications. Liberians live their lives in close community and they like it that way. There is a togetherness to Liberian life that is difficult to even explain. I have never heard a Liberian complain about lack of "personal space," but I have seen elderly women practically start to cry when they heard that my baby slept in a wicker bassinet next to my bed rather than in bed with me.

Obtaining water is complicated and basic sanitation is a problem in many Liberian homes. While Monrovia has a water system, it is not always turned on. And even when it is working, many people have no access to it. Instead they draw their water from wells. Consequently for many people it is an arduous process to get water into their homes. Houses without Western-style bathrooms have no indoor toilet. A shared outhouse or whatever available scrap of private space takes its place. All that being said, Liberians are scrupulously clean. Morning and evening they take scalding hot bucket baths. Most often this is done in a bathhouse, which is a small, semi-permanent enclosure in the yard.

Even eating is complicated. Unlike our grocery stores with their broad aisles of goods making them one-stop shopping experiences, shopping in Liberia involves multiple interactions with people in bustling, outdoor settings. To buy rice, people go to one vendor. The onions, bouillon cubes and salt may come from another, while the vegetables for the sauce come from a third. Most people go to the market every day. They cook their food outdoors and then sit in a circle and eat from a common bowl. The very real need for food each day and the very real difficulty of obtaining it makes it impossible for most people to stay isolated, much less quarantined, without the cooperation of people leading equally difficult and complicated lives.

Transportation is also complicated. Only the wealthier own a car and most of those are used for a taxi service business rather than as a family vehicle. Yellow taxis are, quite literally, everywhere in the city. If a contagious person on his way to a treatment center either vomits or has an episode of diarrhea while in a taxi, unless a proper clean-up takes place, the next customer will be endangered.

Most complicated of all is contact tracing, the process of finding and interviewing those who may have had exposure to the virus. In the West contact tracing is relatively simple. Directories give home phone numbers. Houses have numbers on the outside and are lined up in neat rows on streets that have names. In Liberia there is no landline phone service and no directory of numbers. Houses are not numbered and many people live in small shacks set amid a labyrinth of other small shacks that are nearly impossible to find without a guide.

Finding those exposed to Ebola through contact tracing is just the first step. For the next twenty-one days the compromised individuals are supposed to be monitored daily for fever and Ebola-like symptoms. If they get Ebola, every contact of theirs is supposed to be traced and monitored for twenty-one days. In the most organized of governmental health systems, the complexity of doing this would be staggering. It seemed impossibly difficult given the lack of resources in Liberia.

Additionally, if contact tracing is going to be effective, it is of utmost importance that all people with Ebola and those who know them tell the truth, the whole truth and nothing but the truth. Unfortunately, Liberia is, at least outwardly, a very accommodating culture. People are taught by example to say what they figure will get them into the least trouble or whatever will most please the questioner.

The ramifications of this mindset for contact tracing Ebola cases is cause for concern. If a person were asked if he had recently attended a funeral and he suspected the "right" answer—the one the tracer was hoping to hear—was no, then "no" would be the answer he might give. If a tracer asked if any family members had recently died and the answer might get the remaining living family members shunned, the temptation to deny any recent deaths would be huge.

The nature of the Ebola virus in combination with the realities of life in Liberia was creating difficult problems with no easy solutions. People in Monrovia knew Ebola patients were at ELWA Hospital, but they did not understand either how lethal the virus was or how necessary it was to protect themselves. I was afraid that unless something changed very soon, things were going to get completely out of control.

Chapter 5:
Our Worst Nightmare

Even as these unpleasant realities of Ebola in Liberia jostled around in my head, I had some much more welcome things to think about as I worked in the ward. Our daughter Heidi was getting married in August and months ago, long before Ebola was even on our radar, we had planned a six-week trip to the States around the wedding.

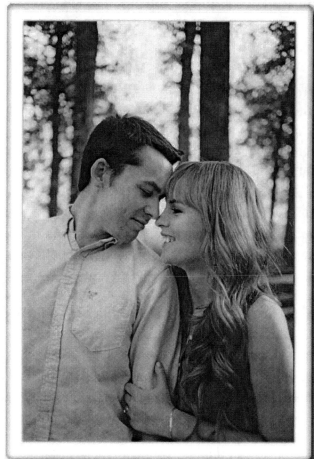

Daniel and Heidi (Image - Rebekah Viola photography)

Mark and I have six children, of whom Heidi is our fourth. She was also the fourth to get married. Born with the gene that teachers love—the passion to do everything assigned as quickly and thoroughly as possible—she had managed to finish her homeschooling requirements for high school graduation at the age of sixteen. She took some college classes online while in Liberia and then started college in the States at seventeen. Now, at nineteen, Heidi had graduated from college and was ready to marry Daniel Markley, who was four years older and shared similar passions and intelligence.

I felt a bit guilty for leaving my spot at the Ebola ward. After the first week of working every night, Mark had jokingly asked if it were possible for someone whose name was *not* Nancy to be trained for the job. Thankfully, there were several people *not* named Nancy willing to be recruited. By the time my family was ready to leave, Eric Buller and Wendy Simpson were working regularly in the ward. Additionally, Samaritan's Purse had new volunteers heading toward West Africa.

The day before our departure, I took Jonah and Jared with me to the ELWA campus. Although I was very busy trying to pull everything together for our trip, I wanted to say goodbye to my friends.

I drove over to the duplex my friend Melanie Ness and her family shared with the Brantlys. Melanie had planned a little event, complete with nail polish, chocolate and hot beverages. By the time I arrived, Amber Brantly and several others were already chatting.

We had a sweet time of fellowship and I felt very privileged to have such good friends with whom to share. The Ebola crisis was on everyone's minds, of course, and much of our talk was about it. We were all keenly aware of the need for God's wisdom and protection for everyone, but most obviously for those working in the ward. In addition to concern for their husbands' safety, Beth Fankhauser and Amber Brantly were dealing with the practical realities of caring for their children and homes while having husbands working in the Ebola ward in addition to their normal doctoring duties.

As Beth, Amber and I talked, it crossed my mind I had an insider's view that could encourage them. Watching Dr. Fankhauser, Dr. Brantly and Dr. Debbie in the ward had touched me deeply and I inevitably cried when I tried to talk about it. While Beth and Amber were home at night with their children, I was with their husbands in the Ebola ward. I knew what they were doing during those long hours.

"Your husbands are doing such a great job," I said to Beth and Amber, who listened attentively. "It's just amazing to watch them work with the patients. They are so gentle and kind. They are being the hands and feet of Christ to these people. It's a really beautiful thing."

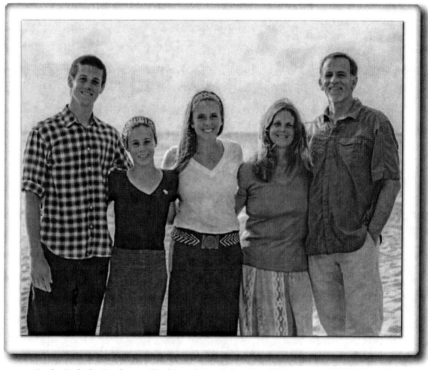

Josh, Bekah, Bethany, Beth and Dr. John Fankhauser at ELWA beach (Image used with permission)

We left Liberia on July 10th as planned. John-Mark, Sara, Audrey and Noah traveled with us. We had a fun night in London and then headed to Minneapolis, our home base in the States. After spending some time with Mark's brother and his wife and getting caught up with our Minnesota relatives, we began a long road trip.

One of our first stops was Pennsylvania. Heidi was living there and wanted to be married in Reading, where Daniel and she would settle after marriage. We wanted to see them, of course, and get to know Heidi's soon-to-be in-laws.

It was on July 26th, while we were eating at the Olive Garden restaurant after just meeting Daniel's parents, that the call came from my son John-Mark saying Dr. Brantly had been diagnosed with Ebola. To say I was shocked was an understatement. Of course I knew it was a possibility that one of us working in the ward could contract the disease, but it had seemed remote. Until it happened. In stunned horror I sobbed and sobbed.

This was awful beyond belief. With such a high mortality rate, what chance did Kent have? I wondered. If Kent were to die, Amber would be left a young widow with children ages five and three to raise by herself. I could only imagine how much she would miss Kent. Could this be happening because of a mistake *I* had made?

Sitting in the restaurant with our new friends, the only response that made any sense was prayer. Timothy Markley led our group, asking for healing for Dr. Brantly, if it were God's will, and peace for us.

Later that night, in the privacy of our hotel room, I searched the internet for any information about what was happening in Liberia. I wanted so badly for this *not* to be happening. But it was. I carefully counted the days since I had last worked in the isolation ward and realized it could not have been a mistake on my part that caused Dr. Brantly's contamination. A huge burden lifted off me.

At midnight a Facebook message from a friend appeared. "This is not public yet, but Nancy Writebol also tested positive for Ebola this evening. We are all pretty shell shocked." Again, tears poured down my face. I gasped out to Mark what had just appeared on my computer screen. This seemed totally surreal. We were so very, very careful. Every single protocol had been followed to the best of our ability. There were no shortcuts taken. Ever.

My mind raced. I had seen Ebola mercilessly ravage and kill. In the weeks that I worked in the ward there had only been one survivor, Gartee, who was young and his illness diagnosed early. While I could begin to imagine that a thirty-three year-old man like Dr. Brantly might have a slim hope of survival, I knew that Nancy was totally exhausted and fifty-nine years old. What possible chance did she have? I felt absolutely sick to think that most likely both of my friends would die the same gruesome deaths I had witnessed in the

Ebola ward. And this would happen very soon. On the other side of the world it was already in the process of happening.

I thought also of David Writebol. He and Nancy had been married for more than forty years and were deeply in love. Nancy charmed him and it showed all over his face. I had seen him stand behind her beaming as she chatted animatedly about her love of spicy food. I knew that if Nancy died he would be devastated.

I could well imagine the reaction of the missionary and Liberian staff in the Ebola ward. There had been many new cases brought to the new and now larger Ebola ward, called ELWA 2, on the campus. Doctors Without Borders (MSF) was creating yet a third ward, which would be called ELWA 3. How heartbroken, confused and upset they must be when, in the middle of this ever-growing Ebola horror, two of those at the very heart of the fight were found to be infected. Even with these baffling diagnoses, they would have to move forward and function professionally and this would take nothing less than absolute trust in God. If the staff collapsed with grief or fear, the patients would be without proper care.

Within hours of their positive diagnoses, Dr. Brantly and Nancy's pictures were all over the news. I was deeply gratified to observe the respect with which my friends were being treated. Through traditional and social media, people were asked to pray for their healing. In my overwhelming sadness, the very thought of all those prayers comforted me.

Eventually I was able to find out what happened on the days surrounding the diagnoses. On Wednesday, July 23rd, Dr. Brantly woke with a slight fever and feeling a bit sick. He assumed he had malaria. He had been working nights in the Ebola ward, which many times swarmed with mosquitoes. He did a blood test for malaria. It came back negative.

Dr. Brantly's temperature rose and he developed a rash. He called Dr. John Fankhauser who, along with Dr. Nathalie McDermott of Samaritan's Purse, went to his house to take a blood sample to check for Ebola. Decked out in full protective gear, the two joked as Dr. Fankhauser drew his blood. Knowing she would worry, Kent had not called Amber, now in Texas with her family. The test came back negative, but Kent knew that early tests were not conclusive.

Soon he was weak and overwhelmed by nausea. He took two more malaria tests that both came back negative. His fever rose to 104.9° F. He began to have diarrhea, so IV fluids were started in his arm. Everyone was hoping it would be dengue fever.

Throughout the week everyone had done their best to keep the situation light, but on Saturday, July 26th, at six in the morning, when Dr. Fankhauser and Dr. Nathalie McDermott again went to Kent's house to do a blood test for Ebola, everyone knew it was no laughing matter. As my friend Bev Kauffeldt waited outside in her PPE to decontaminate the doctors when they were ready to leave the house, she wondered if it were possible for the horrible week-end—multiple deaths in the ward, local youths threatening to burn down the new Ebola ward being erected on the ELWA campus, and an attack on a group of Ebola-fighting Samaritan's Purse workers in the interior—to get worse.

But it did get worse. When the test results came back, Samaritan Purse's disaster response team leader, Dr. Lance Plyler, came to Kent's bedroom window with the bad news. "Kent, buddy, we have your test results. I am really sorry to tell you that it's positive for Ebola."

With Dr. Fankhauser, who had spent a large portion of the day with him, near his side, Kent called Amber. It was afternoon in Abilene, Texas, where Amber had travelled for her brother's wedding. She had spent the day at her parents' house, feeling sick with worry. She separated herself from the family for privacy when Kent called. Kent broke the bad news. Both she and Kent knew how Ebola usually ended—with death. "I'm sorry. I'm so, so sorry." Amber said over and over as she cried.

It was on her birthday, Tuesday, July 22nd, that Nancy Writebol started feeling sick. Like Dr. Brantly, she also assumed it was malaria. When she tested positive she began the treatment. When she did not get any better and continued to run a fever, the same team who drew blood from Dr. Brantly drew her blood as well. Nancy got the news about her test results at the same time she found out about Dr. Brantly's diagnosis. David shared the news with her in the privacy of their bedroom where she had been resting. He simply said, "Nancy, Kent has Ebola. And you do too."

When David reached out to hug her, Nancy stopped him. "David, don't. Just don't. It's going to be okay," she said.

The decision was made that both Kent and Nancy would stay in their respective houses. Along with recently arrived Samaritan's Purse nurses, Dr. Fankhauser would care for Dr. Brantly and Dr. Debbie for Nancy. Of course, as was everything with Ebola, it would be very complicated. The doctors and nurses would have to be de-contaminated at the doorways of their houses and the used PPEs bagged and carefully carried away.

My heart ached for my friends and their families. David would not be able to be with Nancy, much less touch her, unless he wore PPE. Although I knew Kent would be relieved that Amber and the children were far from the threat of Ebola, he could not help but be lonely for them.

Once I got over the initial shock, I could talk about the diagnoses without crying. I understood there was no choice but to trust God with the outcome. I knew God would give my friends serving Kent and Nancy the strength they needed for the task and I also knew, while both wanted to live, Kent and Nancy were both willing to die if that is what would bring God the most glory.

Chapter 6:
West Point

August 16th, 2014, Heidi and Daniel's wedding day, dawned warm and beautiful. Our entire family had gathered—Mark and I, our six children, the spouses of the three who were married, and the four grandchildren—for this most precious of occasions. My heart swelled with pride as a beautiful Heidi was ushered down the aisle on Mark's arm.

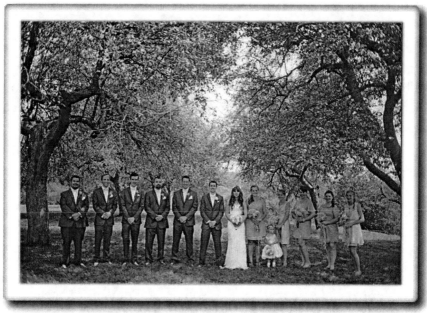

Daniel and Heidi's wedding party (Image - Rebekah Viola photography)

After the wedding and the reception that followed, we returned to our motel room elated yet exhausted. As I uploaded the myriad of pictures I had taken, I opened up my Facebook account. A linked article stopped me cold. It read, "Mob Destroys Ebola Center In Liberia Two Days After It Opens."[1] I knew this was going to be really bad.

In 2005, while still recovering from the Civil War, Ellen Johnson-Sirleaf, known locally as "Ma Ellen," won the country's presidential election. She had a distinct advantage—she did not look like a warlord. After nearly fifteen years, electricity and running water were restored to parts of Monrovia. The horrible roads were repaired. Best of all, there was once again a feeling of stability in Liberia.

But it did not come without a price for some. During the war, a huge number of people displaced from their upcountry homes had settled in Monrovia. They lived in abandoned houses and multi-storied unfinished buildings, as well as tiny shacks they put together with old roofing sheets. So desperate were they to be out of rebel-controlled areas, they would put up with deplorable living conditions.

As the country became more stable, squatters were evicted from their borrowed homes. Still unwilling or unable to return to the interior, they joined the tens of thousands already living in West Point, Liberia's largest slum. Now, all these years later, the half-mile long peninsula remained home to more than fifty thousand people. The vast majority of its residents lived in tiny, unplumbed shacks.

On this small but heavily-populated peninsula, an Ebola isolation center was created in an empty school building. Cooking supplies, mattresses and bedding were supplied to people who had been exposed to Ebola—some symptomatic and some not. Two days into its operation, a woman brought food for her husband and son. When she was not allowed to enter the facility, she became upset. West Point residents helped her relatives crawl over a wall and leave.

A crowd gathered and got into an uproar. Some were openly saying there was no such thing as Ebola and insisting that those who were sick were suffering from malaria. Others who believed Ebola was real were complaining that the government had brought suspected victims from other areas of the city into West Point. No doubt

---

[1] http://www.buzzfeed.com/jinamoore/two-days-after-it-opens-mob-destroys-ebola-center-in-liberia accessed October 3, 2014

fearing how this was going to end, those in quarantine fled from the Ebola isolation center. Some were seen leaving West Point.

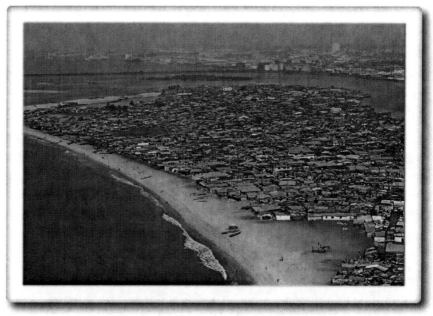

West Point (Image - Bethany Fankhauser)

As the quarantined people left, the looting began. Mattresses and sheets stained with blood and feces were carried through muddy alleyways and away from the isolation center. Riot police and soldiers were sent in. Clashes broke out and people starting throwing rocks. Officers ordered residents indoors.

When the news hit the broader population that the city's most populous slum had just shot out seventeen potential health time bombs, the implications rocked the capital city. President Ellen Johnson-Sirleaf announced a lockdown. No one was to leave West Point for twenty-one days. Roadblocks made of scrap wood and barbed wire were hastily erected. The police and the military manned them.

The implementation of the quarantine was sudden and it caught people off guard. In fact, those visiting West Point found themselves detained alongside those who lived there. People were afraid and upset. But tensions rose to the next level when a West Point government commissioner was allowed to return to the cordoned-off district to bring her children out. West Point residents and those trapped in with them were furious. Hundreds of angry people, many of them young men, marched toward a security checkpoint, pelting stones.

The security forces were overwhelmed. Afraid of touching people and risking Ebola, members of the Armed Forces of Liberia started shooting up into the air. In the bedlam a fifteen year-old boy was shot in one leg and sustained a deep laceration on the other. His wounds proved to be fatal. The president announced a curfew from nine in the evening until six in the morning for the city.[2]

Things quieted down, but underneath the restored calm was deep angst. The people were not only caught unaware, they had been caught unprepared. There were not enough supplies inside the quarantined area to go around and the price of what was there rose immediately. The president, in response, promised food would be brought to them.

We watched all of this with alarm through news articles coming out of Liberia. Because of our years in refugee work, we understood the complicated dynamics and I was truly afraid for Liberia in general and West Point in particular. Gripped by paranoia and suspicion and with an uncertain number of hidden Ebola cases, the Liberian people and their government leaders were poised to become the worst version of themselves.

Even while the Ebola crisis was small, the country seemed overwhelmed and unprepared. As the epidemic grew and more lives were affected, the too-little-too-late response of the government was obvious to even Ma Ellen's most ardent supporters.

Various governments from around the world were giving huge amounts of money to fight Ebola. The Liberian government had already taken multiple hits for the questionable way it had handled the funds. Large sums of money disappeared with little to show for it.[3] Basic needs of patients in the various wards were unmet and staff salaries unpaid. In some locations medical staff were refusing to work because they were not provided even basic protective

---

[2] http://www.foxnews.com/health/2014/08/19/liberia-president-declares-ebola-curfew/

[3] http://www.frontpageafricaonline.com/index.php/politic/3048-us-5m-mystery-what-really-happened-to-ebola-money accessed Oct. 3, 2014

equipment.[4]

Cynicism of the government was not uncommon and many were convinced the whole Ebola crisis was nothing but a moneymaking scheme fabricated to enrich those in power. When the government intervened using both the police and the army, many reacted negatively or even violently because they assumed those in authority were, yet again, out to enrich themselves at the expense of the common man. The President of Liberia was in the middle of a public relations nightmare.

The quarantine for West Point was lifted on Saturday August 30th after just ten days. While President Ellen Johnson-Sirleaf declared it a success, I could not see what it had accomplished. Rejoicing people who misunderstood the purpose of the quarantine in the first place, now misunderstood why it had been lifted. Locals were saying the government had found no Ebola in West Point.

---

[4] http://www.theguardian.com/world/2014/sep/02/ebola-liberian-nurses-strike-lack-protective-equipment accessed Oct. 3, 2014

Chapter 7:
A Present Linked to a Past

Dozens of news articles were being posted on the internet each day about Ebola. While many repeated the same basic information about Ebola itself, I sensed other writers were trying to understand if Liberia's unique past had anything to do with her most unfortunate present.

Because it was so intrinsically tied to that of the United States, I have always found Liberia's history fascinating. The Portuguese began exploring West Africa for the purposes of trade in the fifteenth century. The Dutch and British soon followed. There were two items of special interest. The first was pepper. The abundance of melegueta pepper caused the Europeans to call present day Liberia's coastline the "Pepper Coast." The second item in high demand was slaves. Sadly, intertribal warfare produced a steady supply.

The first Africans arrived in North America with Europeans in 1619 as indentured servants. As the decades passed, laws changed to allow slavery. Slaves were brought by the shipload under inhumane conditions to be sold in markets for use as house servants, artisans, craftsmen and field hands.

By the time the colonists proclaimed their independence from Britain in 1776, slavery was entrenched in American society. The founders of the United States of America asserted in the Declaration of Independence the self-evident truth that "...all men are created equal." Unfortunately it was not self-evident to the founders that those of African descent were created equal as well.

There were always some U.S. citizens who were against slavery and as time passed their numbers grew—especially in the northern States. The southern States, with their expanding cotton industry, were increasingly dependent on slave labor.

In 1807, as a result of William Wilberforce's efforts, England's Atlantic slave trade was abolished when "An Act for the Abolition of the Slave Trade" was passed in their Parliament. The same year a similar law was passed in the United States. The "Act Prohibiting Importation of Slaves" made it illegal for anyone to use the Atlantic Ocean to traffic slaves. It did not, however, prohibit internal slave trading and the huge domestic slave industry continued unabated.

Just as there were increasing numbers of African-American people enslaved, there were also increasing numbers that were free. Some of the free were the descendants of the original indentured servants. Others had been freed as masters converted to abolitionist ideals. Children of freed slaves were, of course, free.

The enslaved population yearned for freedom. At the turn of the century a slave named Gabriel changed the course of history. Gabriel lived in Virginia and was regularly hired out as a blacksmith with the monetary benefits going to his master, Thomas Prosser. Desperate for freedom, on August 30th, 1800, Gabriel planned to lead a group of slaves in an attack on Richmond. When slave owners became suspicious, the state militia was called. Gabriel managed to escape, but was later spotted and turned in by another slave for a reward the state offered. Gabriel and twenty-four others were hung.

Even though this rebellion was over almost before it began, it highlighted the underlying potential for violence. Nearly forty percent of Virginia's population were slaves and the thought of a successful rebellion deeply frightened the white population. People feared the disquieting influence freed Blacks had on the enslaved population. Additionally, because proponents of slavery had gone to great lengths to convince the public there was something inherently different and inferior about black-skinned people, many Whites did not want to see them become equals either in society or under the law. Still others feared jobs going to non-whites or the possibility of increased crime.

In 1816, the American Colonization Society, also known as The Society for the Colonization of Free People of Color of America, was formed. The group was composed of both abolitionists and nonabolitionists. Their goal was to "repatriate" people of African descent to their homeland.

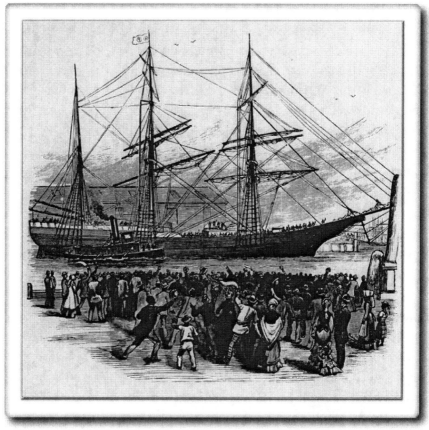

Sketch of ship leaving New York City headed to Liberia (Image - public domain)

In 1821 the society sent its first shipload of eighty-six immigrants to Sherbro Island in Sierra Leone. The swampy, unhealthy conditions were so formidable that within three weeks twenty-two settlers and three society representatives were dead. The remaining settlers were desperate to relocate and in 1822 a representative of the society was sent to purchase land farther down the coast.

After searching for a hospitable location, the representative and a naval officer began negotiations with tribal leaders in the Cape Mesurado area. These leaders were not enthusiastic about forfeiting their land to strangers, but with a bit of persuasion—some say at gunpoint—they finally agreed to give up a strip of coastal land in exchange for approximately three hundred dollars worth of goods.

The surviving colonists moved to Cape Mesurado, named their colony Christopolis, and tried to make it home.

The new colonists did not appreciate being governed by the society's white representative and some took up arms. The representative fled. The society sent another representative to negotiate and eventually a consensus was reached. Power would officially remain with the society, but the immigrants would have day-by-day control. The settlement was renamed Monrovia after U.S. President James Monroe, a big supporter of the project, and the colony as a whole was called Liberia.

The American Colonization Society, with the support of the United States government, sent more than 18,000 immigrants to Liberia. Several southern states, eager to be rid of freed blacks and their worrisome influence on the enslaved population, formed their own societies and sent still more. The new settlers brought with them the housing and clothing styles of the antebellum South.

Taxation was a major source of revenue for the new commonwealth. Traders, both European and indigenous, were taxed. The British were unhappy with this arrangement and announced they did not recognize the authority of the American Colonization Society to levy taxes. The colonists decided they needed to become an independent nation with full taxing authority if they were going to survive. In 1847 the Republic of Liberia was founded.

While the white founders of the American Colonization Society thought of Africa as the true homeland of freed slaves, the truth was that the United States was their homeland and its culture what they knew. The Americo-Liberians, the name given to those who came from the United States, thought they had little or nothing in common with the indigenous people of Liberia. The indigenous people spoke their tribal languages and wore very different clothing. The Americo-Liberians called them "savages" and did not consider it wrong to take their land and resources. In this new society where the lighter the skin the better, strict rules were put in place to make sure the classes stayed separate. The indigenous people were not educated. They were not even allowed to vote.

One of the goals of the American Colonization Society was to use repatriation as a means of Christian evangelism. Many of the indigenous people, whose religious practices harkened back to a time no one could even remember, did not oppose adding the new-comers' tradition of Christianity to their spiritual mix. In the same way those who wanted to succeed in this new environment adopted the Americo-Liberians' English language, the indigenous people in large numbers joined churches and immersed themselves in church activities. They changed their names to Western names—often biblical ones—and basically did whatever they could to become what the Americo-Liberians and they themselves now considered "civilized."

Because of the disparity in opportunity between the Americo-Liberians, who made up less than five percent of the population, and the indigenous people, tension always simmered beneath the surface. Despite that, for more than one hundred and thirty years after becoming independent, Liberia had a relatively stable government—always under the leadership of an Americo-Liberian.

All of that changed in 1980 when Samuel K. Doe, a sergeant in the Liberian army and a member of the indigenous Krahn tribal group, led a bloody coup that unseated Americo-Liberian President William Tolbert. Cabinet members were tied to poles on the beautiful Atlantic Ocean shoreline near the presidential mansion and shot. When government workers were imprisoned or worse, a mass exodus of the Americo-Liberian elite began, shaking up the entire power structure of the country.

Although poorly educated and completely ill-suited for the job, Doe declared himself Liberia's ruling head. Liberia and its economy began a downward spiral. Shortly before we had arrived in Liberia in 1986, a man of the Gio (Dan) tribe named Thomas Quiwonkpa made several coup attempts, the last one resulting in his death. Doe's resultant anger was against not just Quiwonkpa, but Quiwonkpa's entire Dan tribe.

Charles Taylor, a Liberian graduate of Bentley College in Massachusetts and a previous Doe employee, saw the tribal tensions and understood how to exploit them. On December 24, 1989, while we were in Wisconsin on our one-year home assignment from Liberia celebrating Christmas with family, Charles Taylor and his band of

National Patriotic Front of Liberia (NPFL) rebels crossed into Liberia from the Ivory Coast's western border and invaded Butuo, a village populated by people from both the Gio and Mano tribes.

The Liberian army, with its high percentage of ethnically Krahn soldiers, rushed to stop the invasion. They brutally attacked the residents of any village whom they claimed had "hosted" the advancing rebels. Husbands and wives were separated as they ran in opposite directions. Children unable to keep up were lost in the chaos. Soldiers threw hundreds of babies into water-filled wells.

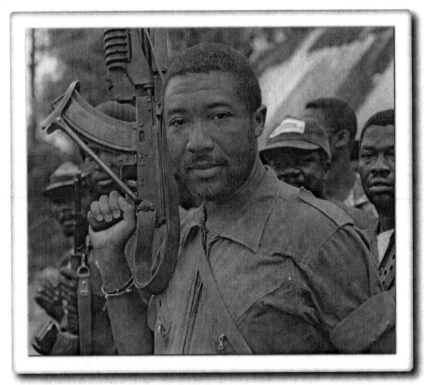

Charles Taylor (Image - public domain)

President Doe's army so mishandled the crisis they actually created an army of Taylor followers in their wake. The invasion and its aftermath began a fourteen year on-again, off-again civil war that claimed hundreds of thousands of lives and displaced and maimed countless more. Newspapers around the world carried the stories, complete with pictures. Rebels posed for journalists in the outfits they wore into battle, including bright pink wigs, graduation gowns and tattered wedding dresses.

Despite his original claim that his only goal was to liberate the country from Doe, after years of war and a long series of unsuccessful peace talks most Liberians concluded the war would not be over until Taylor was president. With campaign slogans that included the now infamous "You killed my ma, you killed my pa, I'll vote for you," Taylor won 1997's presidential election in a landslide.

After only months in office and in spite of unspeakable atrocities against the Liberian people, it was for crimes against humanity in Sierra Leone that Taylor finally faced official accusations. The government of Sierra Leone, Liberia's neighbor, accused Taylor of fueling and financing their own civil war that left tens of thousands of its citizens dead and countless more maimed and mutilated.

Taylor's enemies were countless, making his constant state of paranoia truly appropriate. Two different groups of rebels fighting Taylor's government were gaining control of more and more of Liberia's interior land. When fighting reached Monrovia yet again, it all proved to be too much for Taylor to overcome. He relinquished the presidency and in 2003 was taken by airplane to a new life in Nigeria where he would be protected, at least for a while, by their government.[1]

Liberia's long nightmare was over at last.

---

[1] Taylor remained in Nigeria until 2006 when Liberia's president Johnson-Sirleaf formally requested his extradition. He then attempted to flee Nigeria but was arrested by Nigerian officials and sent to Liberia, who turned him over to U.N. soldiers. They brought him to Sierra Leone to stand trial for war crimes against the people of Sierra Leone. To keep from destabilizing Sierra Leone he was moved to the Penitentiary Institution at the Hague, Netherlands. His trial before the International Criminal Court, lasting almost six years, was held in Leidschendam, Netherlands. He eventually was found guilty in April, 2012, on eleven counts of "aiding and abetting" war crimes and crimes against humanity, sentenced to fifty years in prison and imprisoned in the United Kingdom. For more information go to http://edition.cnn.com/2012/05/30/world/africa/netherlands-taylor-sentencing/index.html and http://en.wikipedia.org/wiki/Charles_Taylor_(Liberian_politician)

Chapter 8:
Witchcraft

As Mark and I scoured the internet, reading every available article about Ebola in Liberia, we read of the dismay of health professionals and news reporters when they discovered many Liberians did not believe Ebola was real. Sadly, Mark and I were not surprised.

Several years ago we spent over a year working almost exclusively with one small church in a Monrovia suburb. Each Sunday for forty-five minutes while Mark taught the men, I taught the women's Sunday school class. My most enthusiastic student was a forty year-old widow named Dorcas, who would literally sit on the edge of her seat, so intent was she on understanding what I was teaching.

One Wednesday evening, during the time allotted to share prayer requests, Dorcas raised her hand. "I need prayer," she said sadly. "I need to separate from my sister. She is a witch. Sometimes she turns into a black cat at night and has even been known to kill babies." Titus, the Bible school student leading the service, nodded and jotted down her request on the piece of paper in front of him.

I was stunned. Had I just heard what I thought I heard? How in the world could my prize student believe a person could turn into a cat? A black cat that kills babies in the night, no less? How could her poor sister defend herself from such an accusation if the proof were simply that somewhere near her was a dead baby? Equally disturbing was the fact that the Bible school student writing down the prayer requests had not said a word to suggest he did not believe the situation to be exactly as Dorcas had stated.

On the way home Mark and I had another one of our "This is worse than we thought" conversations. We acknowledged that despite how long we had worked among the Liberians, we constantly underestimated the extent to which animism, the belief that the seen world is animated by unseen spiritual forces, permeated their culture.

Liberia has to be one of the most religious countries in the world. According to the nation's 2008 census, its population of about four million claims to be eighty-five percent Christian and twelve percent Muslim.[1] In Monrovia there seems to be a church on every corner and Liberians begin everything from business meetings to birthday parties in prayer. However, they also embrace an animistic worldview.

Until we came to Liberia we rarely thought about worldview, that philosophy of life or understanding of the world that creates the "glasses" through which a person looks at and interprets the world around him. Once in Liberia, however, we were constantly confronted with beliefs and cultural traditions very different from our own, forcing us to give serious thought to this issue.

Liberia's worldview realities go back to the early settlers and those first important years. While Colonization Society representatives hoped the immigrants would bring the gospel to the indigenous people, most settlers were not equipped for this ambitious task. Many of the immigrants practiced their Christian faith alongside deeply-held folk beliefs inherited from their African ancestors. The thoroughly animistic beliefs and practices of the indigenous people would eventually have an enormous impact on the worldview of the settlers as these two groups interacted together. Rather than turning from animism to a biblical worldview, many Liberians combined these two opposing belief systems to create their own syncretistic version of the Christian faith.

In Liberia the art of managing and manipulating the spiritual forces is commonly known as "witchcraft" and we knew our knowledge of it barely scratched the surface. For years Mark had been waiting either to understand it enough to speak intelligently or for someone more qualified to step up to the plate and teach it for him. That Wednesday evening his procrastination came to an abrupt halt.

---

[1] http://monrovia.usembassy.gov/reports/irfr.html

No matter how much Mark disliked stepping into an area of teaching for which he felt so ill-prepared, he realized no one else was going to come to *that* church and teach Dorcas and Titus what they needed to know to be set free from their fear and confusion. Like it or not, the job was his.

Mark spent the next weeks preparing a series of lessons he entitled, "Witchcraft and the Bible." Week by week he unfolded biblical truths during the Sunday school hour, hoping at least a few in the church would understand the extent to which animism inappropriately dominated their worldview. He eventually took his teaching about animism on the road, demystifying Liberia's witchcraft for larger audiences. At various conferences, seminars and church meetings, he taught what he was starting to understand more clearly.

In African Traditional Religion, the spirits of the dead are believed to play an active role in the lives of the living. Those who hold to these beliefs honor their ancestors through libations and offerings of rice meal, cola nuts and, at times, animal sacrifices. In some areas, the tombs of respected elders are built against the outside walls of houses to ensure that their spirits do not wander far from the village. It is believed that the ancestors intercede to the creator god on behalf of the living for health and good harvests. Failure to honor the ancestors can result in the cessation of their intercession or even personal attacks on the living.

African Traditional Religion also teaches that there are impersonal spiritual forces that can cause great harm if not managed properly. While Westerners think of a "witch" as an ugly, green-faced woman in a pointed black hat and robe, in Liberian English a *witch* is a curse or a spirit that can possess a person. It is believed this spirit can operate independently of the possessed person's body, leaving it at night to harm people by the destruction of property or the consumption of their souls.

It is common knowledge in Liberia that rivers, forests and mountains are home to a large variety of spirit beings. There are the great forest spirits, who are central to the activities of the secretive Poro and Sande initiation societies. Lurking in the muddy rivers are dangerous aquatic spirits like the "neegee," who grab unsuspecting victims from the shore and drown them. Perhaps most common are the "jina," who come in all shapes and sizes including one-footed and one-eyed varieties. Similar to the "jina" are the forest dwarfs who are characterized by backwards-pointing feet and superhuman strength.

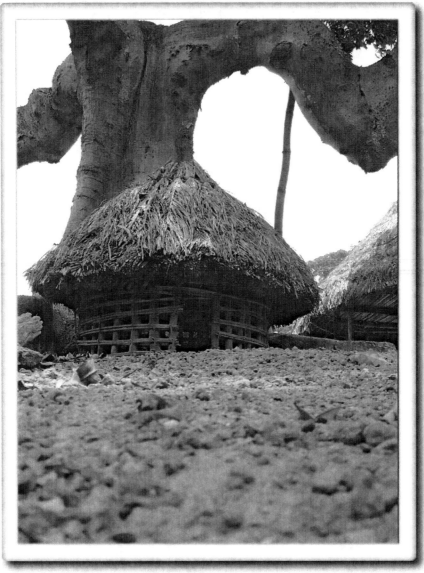

A "spirit house" built at the base of a kapok tree, believed to be the abode of spirits, over a small rock where offerings are laid (Image - John-Mark Sheppard)

These creatures are not considered evil, but simply powerful and potentially dangerous. If not properly recognized and appeased through offerings and sacrifices, these spirits can wreak havoc. Witchcraft is an attempt to control these capricious spirits in order to bring about prosperity or cause harm to one's enemies.

Witchcraft played a huge part in Liberia's civil war. Human sacrifice and cannibalism, practiced by the various rebel factions, were thought to be a means of gaining spiritual power, thus ensuring victory in battle. The weird wigs and crazy outfits in which they ran to battle were worn to protect identities from the spirits who wished to harm them.

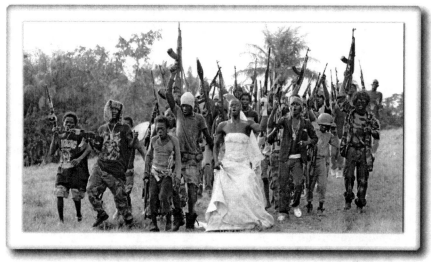

Rebels going into battle - Reenactment from "Johnny Mad Dog"
(Image - public domain)

In the same way Westerners tend to seek a rational or logical explanation for events, most West Africans seek a spiritual explanation. While the average Liberian would not go to a "juju man" to cast a spell on his enemies, many live in daily fear that others will "witch" them. Sadly, fear of witchcraft creates a culture of fatalistic resignation. Why work hard in your business if someone may "witch" you and make it fail no matter what you do? Why build a big house if some jealous person is just going to "witch" you and make you sick so you never can enjoy it? If personal poverty is a result of witchcraft, applying money-management skills is pointless. If a curse is the root of marriage problems, counseling will not help at all.

To the vast majority of Liberians, death is believed to be ultimately the result of a spiritual attack. When people die, even elderly people, much thought goes into deciding who is to blame. Who "witched" the deceased? Sadly, in most churches in Liberia these beliefs are never challenged. In many churches the pastor presents himself as a powerful "Man of God" with the power to protect his congregants against these malevolent forces—if, of course, they will demonstrate their faith by sowing "seed money" into his ministry.

Witchcraft pervades every aspect of the Liberian culture and the countries around it. Darrow Miller in *Discipling Nations: The Power of Truth to Transform Cultures,* tells of the experience of a Peace Corps worker in Sierra Leone, Liberia's neighbor and an epicenter of the Ebola drama.

> Josie Kornegay worked as a Peace Corps nurse for the Serabu Mission Hospital in the Bo District of Sierra Leone, West Africa. She had just finished teaching a microbiology course for ten local nursing students. All of them had worked hard, mastered the information, and demonstrated knowledge of the viruses, bacteria, and other microscopic organisms that cause disease. After the final exam, one student raised her hand and said. "Miss, I know that you taught us about polio, but do you want to know how people really get it?"
>
> Her heart sinking, Josie asked. "How?"
>
> "It's the witches!" her student said. "They are invisible. They fly around at night and bite people's backs!"
>
> Josie told me later, "At that moment with a heaviness of heart, I realized that as far as the Sierra Leonean students were concerned, I didn't know what I was talking about. Their grandmothers had taught them that witches were real and microorganisms were what white people believed in."[2]

The practical ramifications of such beliefs are overwhelming. If Liberians do not believe AIDS is a real disease but instead just another manifestation of a spiritual attack, they will not protect themselves appropriately. If malaria and dysentery are a result of a jealous neighbor's "witching," then protection against mosquitos and pure drinking water are not prioritized. When mothers die in childbirth or children are born handicapped, it is the children themselves who are often diagnosed by a "sandcutter" (diviner) as being the

---

[2] Darrow L. Miller, *Discipling Nations*, (Seattle: YWAM Publishing, 2001), 33.

cause of the problem. Instead of being seen as innocent babies, they are viewed as potential threats.

Liberians see themselves as having three choices when sick. First, self-medicate. A variety of drugs and herbs are available without prescription both in small shops and from street vendors. Second, they can go to a clinic for Western medical treatment. While these imported drugs and treatments may help in some cases, they are insufficient to treat ailments that are perceived as originating in the spirit world. For these a third option is necessary. A traditional healer.

When I read an "herbalist" claimed to have the power to heal Ebola and her resulting death was responsible for the spread of Ebola from Guinea to Sierra Leone, it made sense to me.[3] Zoe (pronounced |zō|), traditional healer, country doctor or herbalist—it was all the same thing. It was the name for the priests or priestesses who conducted healing rituals in the "sick bush."

The sick bush is a secret enclosure in the forest where these traditional healers practice what is known as "African science." Pronounced "African sign," it is a common Liberian term that positively compares the traditional African "spiritual" sources of power with the power of Western science.

Zoes are necessary both to stop evil and to give power to those willing to pay the price to achieve it. Many Liberians believe the power of the zoe's "medicine" (charms, incantations, etc.) to be stronger than any drug found in a pharmacy. A zoe can cure sickness unknown to Western medicine. He can protect from the spirit of a dead grandmother who is disturbing a marriage. He can even catch the witch that is trying to eat a baby's soul. To have no access to such services is to be left completely vulnerable.

It is assumed Westerners cannot understand this African science. When "book people," which includes all Westerners, say one thing and the zoes say another, often outward nods of agreement will be given to the learned outsiders, but inward allegiance still goes to the zoe. This is especially true if individuals have been to the "bush

---

[3] http://www.ibtimes.co.uk/ebola-outbreak-womans-healing-powers-claim-caused -deadly-virus-spread-guinea-1461906

schools," a function of the traditional power associations in which males are initiated into the Poro society and females into the Sande society.

About half of Liberian tribal groups observe these traditions in some form. Adolescents are secluded in secret camps for a period of several weeks to several months where they are taught basic life skills and instructed in society matters. In the Poro society, male initiates are marked with ritual scars on their faces or backs. In the Sande bush girls undergo female genital mutilation (FGM), commonly called "female circumcision." Upon completion, graduates are given a new name and presented to their families as adults. At this point they are privy to secrets, the powerful knowledge hidden from the general public but made known to those who have joined one of the "secret societies."

By the time they reach adulthood, the average Liberians' belief in the power of the spirit world is real and often consuming. Much time and mental energy is spent worrying about invisible attacks from witches, jinas and ancestral spirits. Great sums of money are spent securing the services of zoes, sandcutters and "Men of God" who have the esoteric knowledge and power to protect their clients from these fearsome spiritual forces

When experts talk of viruses to someone with an animistic worldview, who has been taught from childhood that sickness is a result of witchcraft, the experts sound at best irrelevant or at worst foolish. As in Guinea and Sierra Leone, when Ebola came to Liberia, many saw it as another example of malevolent spirits preying on them. The way to stop the attack was through the power of "African science" with the correct herbs, talismans or incantations.

Chapter 9:
"God Save Our State"

The British Air flight we had scheduled to take us home to Liberia after Heidi's wedding was cancelled. Other airlines followed suit. The Peace Corp pulled their 340 volunteers out of West Africa. Foreign businessmen and women were leaving and those airlines still flying out of Liberia were full of whoever had the means and opportunity to escape.

We were not sure what to do. Our Liberian friends were calling us, advising us to delay our return. Our mission agency was doing the same. Six year-old Jonah was loving the excitement of traveling in the United States and did not mind staying longer, but it was tougher for Jared who felt displaced and, unlike Jonah, understood fully what was going on in Liberia.

Mark's brother Steve and his wife Dawn had opened their home in Elk River, Minnesota, to us. Their six boys were young adults and out of the home at the perfect time for us to take over the space they vacated.

The media outlets were full of stories of Ebola's march through Liberia. At the end of July Liberia's land borders were closed to keep the virus from spreading. President Ellen Johnson-Sirleaf declared a ninety-day state of emergency beginning August 6th. She requested residents observe three days of fasting and praying. In closing her presidential address Ma Ellen said, "God save our state." I could not imagine a more fitting closing.

Life for everyone changed. Restrictions were put on public gatherings. Schools were closed, as were all crowd-drawing events. Church gatherings were an exception to the rule. "Ebola buckets" of chlorinated water sat outside of offices, restaurants, hotels and stores; security guards made sure people used them. Temperatures were taken before entering government offices with the resulting number pinned on to clothing. Radio messages, signs and songs encouraged people to recognize Ebola was real and to take precautions. "Kick Ebola Out" trended on social media and the "No New Infections" hashtag became popular.

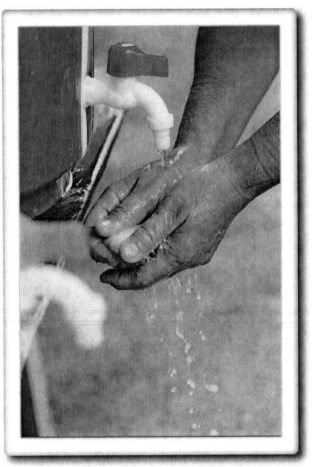

Stores quickly sold out of medical gloves. Pharmacies sold out of medicines as enterprising marketers realized drugs could be hawked on the streets at highly inflated prices.

(Image - Bethany Fankhauser)

The Liberian government banned bush meat, a major source of both income and protein to many. Research was showing that fruit dropped by a bat could potentially be eaten by another animal that could in turn become a carrier.

A serious food crisis was looming. It was known that some farmers were leaving their crops unharvested as they fled Ebola-stricken areas. What was not always so clear was whether the claimed shortages of food and goods were real or if vendors were simply taking advantage of the Ebola crisis to hike their prices.

With the departure of those who would rent the best apartments and buy the most food, clothes and services, many were losing their primary sources of income. Those suffering most were the families who lost their breadwinners to Ebola. Already in mourning and often ostracized because of their potential contact with the virus, these families now faced starvation.

The Liberian Ministry of Defense launched "Operation White Shield," whose goal was to quarantine people in certain regions where Ebola was found. The Armed Forces of Liberia set up and guarded checkpoints—ropes spread across roads—to keep people either in or out of designated areas. While relief organizations were doing their best to provide food to the impacted areas, those in quarantine who were overlooked faced a serious dilemma. If they stayed and respected the quarantine, they went hungry. If they escaped through a jungle path or another route, they were not honoring the intent of the quarantine.

I remained deeply concerned for Dr. Brantly and Nancy Writebol in Liberia. I knew they were walking through a very dark valley. They were too weak and sick to care for themselves and those who served them had to be in Tyvek® suits. That being said, I knew beyond any doubt that none of their colleagues would resent the difficulty of the care. They would consider it a privilege.

Everyone knew prayer for Dr. Brantly and Nancy was absolutely vital. In Monrovia, outside of Kent and Nancy's houses, missionaries and Liberian staff members prayed in a circle holding hands. Countless people around the world were hearing of Kent and Nancy's plight and praying as well.

Kent's condition was deteriorating. With high fevers, chills and racing heart, his body began to shake and his breathing was labored. His temperature remained high despite all attempts to bring it down. He could tell he had fluid in his lungs. He felt hot, nauseated and weak.

Kent and Amber talked daily on Skype. As he deteriorated, Amber wondered each morning if Kent would still be alive. With his bloody diarrhea and vomit, high temperature, shaking body, labored breathing, racing heart and red eyes, he was extremely sick. Disconcertingly, Kent had never treated a patient with his advanced symptoms who survived.

With nothing to do but lie in bed, both Kent and Nancy had time to evaluate what had happened. How had they been exposed? While Kent thought that perhaps he had been compromised in the emergency room where cases were triaged, Nancy had no clue how she was exposed. Certainly nothing was obvious.

As the situation became more desperate, Dr. Debbie, Dr. Fankhauser and Dr. Plyler tried to do anything and everything that might possibly help. Both Kent and Nancy received blood from some local friends in hopes it could make a difference.

The family of our young survivor was contacted. Because they were so very grateful for what Dr. Brantly had done in helping to save his life, Gartee's family was happy to allow him to give blood. Gartee's plasma, full of antibodies, could possibly strengthen Kent and help his body fight the disease.

The news media was thrilled with this story. Because Gartee was there when I worked, I knew exactly who was being spoken of and to even think of it brought tears to my eyes. This young boy had been a sweetheart in the ward, always cooperative and never complaining. It had been wonderful when he had been allowed to go home. No one expected to see him again, certainly not in such a capacity.

Phones rang around the world as Dr. Brantly and Nancy's friends and colleagues desperately tried to gain access to experimental treatments. On Thursday, July 31st, the phone calls paid off. They found a single three-dose treatment of the experimental drug ZMapp[1] in Sierra Leone. While it had worked on monkeys, it had yet to be tested on humans.

The ZMapp lay frozen in a Styrofoam container. It was driven to the border of Guinea and brought into Liberia by canoe. Then it was flown to Monrovia by a Samaritan's Purse airplane.

---

[1] ZMapp is an experimental drug created by Mapp Biopharmaceutical, Inc. for the treatment of Ebola patients. For more information, see http://www.mappbio.com/

Since it seemed she was more ill than he, Kent insisted Nancy receive the ZMapp, which consisted of three doses. However, after the first dose of ZMapp was taken out of the container and placed under Nancy's arm to thaw, Kent's condition deteriorated significantly. At Dr. Plyler's suggestion, Kent agreed to split the treatment with Nancy—he receiving the first dose and the remaining two doses went to Nancy.[2]

After receiving the ZMapp Kent shook violently for thirty minutes. After an hour his rash started to fade. He was able to walk to the bathroom. Kent had not been out of bed for the last day and a half, so this was an encouraging sign. Nancy did not respond as positively.

While all this was going on, I often thought of an experience our family had in 2009 when our daughter Melodie, severely ill with Salmonella poisoning and malaria, was medically evacuated to Europe in a small air ambulance. I knew Kent and Nancy needed a similar evacuation.

Franklin Graham, the president of Samaritan's Purse, was thinking the same way. Dr. Brantly was in Liberia under SP's sponsorship and now he was in real danger of dying. Mr. Graham was determined that every possible chance of survival be given. His determination paid off when he located a long-range business jet with an isolation pod and the necessary clearances were secured.

The decision was made to transport Kent first. The medical charter left from Cartersville, Georgia, on Thursday evening, July 31st. It returned from Liberia with Dr. Brantly at 11:20 a.m. on August 2nd to Dobbins Air Force Base in Atlanta. For the entire trip Kent had been in an isolation pod dressed in a Tyvek® suit. He communicated with the others in the airplane with a walkie-talkie.

An excited American media flew in helicopters overhead following the ambulance carrying Kent from the airfield to Emory University Hospital. The back doors of the vehicle opened and, to my surprise and delight, Kent stepped out of the ambulance and walked slowly into the hospital leaning on a Tyvek®-suit clad paramedic. No

---

[2] http://www.haventoday.org/all-about-jesus-blog/saving-kent-brantly-an-interview-with-dr-lance-plyler-163.html

one had expected him to be able to walk into the hospital.

Emory University Hospital was well prepared to receive Kent. It was one of four hospitals in the U.S. with the capacity to deal with Ebola patients. A team of more than one hundred staff members had been training for years for this moment. All were volunteers—some even giving up vacations to help with Kent's care.

Dr. Brantly's family was euphoric when they saw him still alive and doing better than they had dared to hope. Amber's statement to the media reflected what all of us who knew Kent and loved Liberia felt. "It was a relief to welcome Kent home today. I spoke with him, and he is glad to be back in the U.S. I am thankful to God for his safe transport and for giving him the strength to walk into the hospital. Please continue praying for Kent and Nancy (Writebol), and please continue praying for the people of Liberia and those who continue to serve them there."[3]

Once settled into the unit, Amber was able to see Kent through glass in a door. He was red eyed and swollen, but alive.

Meanwhile Nancy was still waiting in Liberia. I was afraid she would not survive until the plane returned to Liberia to get her. When I heard, two days after Kent arrived at Emory, that she was in the air, my hopes for her survival soared. The flight landed at Dobbins Air Force Base in Atlanta on Tuesday, August 5th. I eagerly watched as reporters in helicopters recorded the police escort of her ambulance through the slow afternoon traffic.

Like Kent, Nancy was in a Tyvek® suit. Unlike him, she was not able to walk into the hospital. Instead she was wheeled in on a stretcher, looking practically mummified in the gear that had kept her isolated during transport.

In the following days the media outlets were hounding Samaritan's Purse and SIM for any tidbit about Dr. Brantly and Nancy and I clung to all of it in fascination. Good news slowly trickled out of Emory. As my friends' health improved, the stories became sources of great encouragement and even some amusement. I had no doubt

---

[3] http://www.reuters.com/article/2014/08/02/us-health-ebola-evacuation-id USKBN0G20D220140802

that if she knew it were happening, Nancy would laugh out loud at the craziness that her asking for a Starbucks coffee was considered newsworthy.

Even after they started to feel better, Nancy and Kent were both still confined to their isolation rooms. However, they were becoming more active. They both wanted showers. Kent played Nerf basketball with some of the nurses. And both were starting to eat again. Pizza for Nancy. Chick-fil-A for Kent.

On August 18th, after being flown from Liberia on a Samaritan's Purse flight, David Writebol made the following statement.

> It has been three weeks since Nancy and I learned of her infection with the Ebola virus. In the ensuing days, we learned much more about the disease than we already knew. We also learned a great deal about the love and compassion of people toward Nancy through the overwhelming outpouring of prayers and well-wishes on our behalf. For this we are truly grateful.
>
> I have completed the 21-day period of precautionary temperature and health monitoring and reporting as mandated by local and state public health authorities, with no symptoms of Ebola Virus Disease. I therefore was cleared to travel to Emory University Hospital to be reunited with Nancy and observe her recovery and return to health. My family and I look forward to her speedy restoration, and we give thanks for continued prayers on her behalf.
>
> I have had the great joy to be able to look through the isolation room glass and see my beautiful wife again. We both placed our hands on opposite sides of the glass, moved with tears to look at each other again. She was standing with her radiant smile, happy beyond words. She is continuing to slowly gain strength, eager for the day when the barriers separating us are set aside, and we can simply hold each other. We prayed together over the intercom, praising our great and mighty God for his goodness to us.[4]

I was thrilled. It seemed God was going to spare the lives of both of my friends.

---

[4] http://simusa.org/content/latest-news/4519/david_writebol_completes_medical_monitoring_period_visits_wife_in_atlanta

Chapter 10:
Exporting Ebola

More and more cases of Ebola were being confirmed in West Africa. The experts' confidence about containment was shattered. Unlike previous outbreaks that occurred in rural, isolated communities, the epicenter of this one was the border region of three countries, all with highly mobile populations. In past outbreaks, experts had been able to cordon off the infected area and prevent further spread of the disease. It was proving difficult to stop Ebola from spreading in crowded cities with motorcycles, cars, taxis and buses moving untold numbers of people in any and all directions.

When speaking of the Ebola outbreak in West Africa, Dr. Steve Monroe, a spokesman for the CDC, said, "This is the largest Ebola outbreak in history and the first in West Africa. It's a rapidly changing situation and we expect there will be more cases in these countries in the coming weeks and months. The response to this outbreak will be more of a marathon than a sprint."[1] Depressing as the words were, I did not doubt them for a moment.

Ebola was on the evening news and people read updates from every possible media outlet. Through all this they witnessed the horrors of what was happening in West Africa and there were differing opinions about everything having to do with Ebola. The one and only thing everyone agreed on was that no one wanted the devastation to reach his or her own country. There was a lot of discussion about how to avoid that nightmare.

---

[1] http://www.cdc.gov/media/releases/2014/t0728-ebola.html

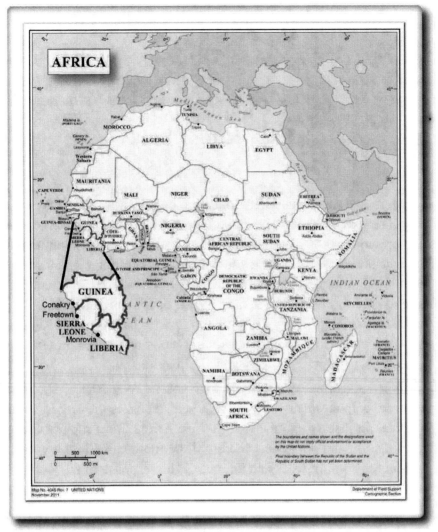

The three countries in West Africa with Ebola epidemics:
Guinea, Sierra Leone and Liberia[2]

Unfortunately sometimes nightmares cannot be avoided. On Sunday, July 20th, Patrick Oliver Sawyer, a 40 year-old Liberian-born American businessman traveled from Liberia to Nigeria. He was noticeably sick. Security cameras caught him lying on the floor at Monrovia's James Spriggs-Payne Airfield as he waited to board his Asky Airlines flight to Nigeria. He vomited in the airplane during

---

[2] Map modified from http://www.un.org/Depts/Cartographic/map/profile/africa.pdf

the flight.

What witnesses to all of this did not know was that Sawyer's twenty-seven year-old sister, Princess Christina Nyennetue, had recently been ill. She had been taken to Monrovia's St. Joseph's Catholic Hospital with heavy bleeding. Her fiancé said she was suffering from a miscarriage. However, when the heavy bleeding continued after a dilatation and curettage (D&C) procedure, the medical staff became suspicious that something else was going on. They wanted her in isolation. Patrick Sawyer insisted his sister be placed in a private room. He changed her clothing, leaving obvious bloodstains on his own clothes and shoes.

Testing was done on Princess's blood. She was found positive for Ebola. She died on July 8th. According to FrontPageAfrica, Patrick Sawyer then sent the following email to his friends:

From: Patrick O. Sawyer <XXX>
Date: Thu, Jul 10, 2014 at 6:09 AM
Subject: Ebola Struck Close to Home
To: Benetta Tarr <XXX>, Benetta Tarr <XXX>
Uria XXX

Dear All,

My junior sister, Miss Princess Christina Nyennetue (Age 27) died on Tuesday July 8th at the St. Joseph Catholic Hospital. At my request, the Ministry of Health agreed to extract blood specimens from her body in search for cause of death and the result just came in this morning...she died of Ebola Disease. Princess was the only girl child of my mother's 5 children... this makes it particularly difficult for us, especially for my mother who lives alone in Southwest Philadelphia . If you Facebook searched my late sister, Princess, you will soon realize that death has cheated a promising young life. Thanks to you all once more for your many messages of condolence and best wishes. Good day.
*Patrick Oliver Sawyer / Head *
ECOWAS NATIONAL OFFICE
*MINISTRY OF FINANCE & DEVELOPMENT PLANNING *[3]

When Sawyer mentioned his sister's death to his employer ArcelorMittal on July 8th, they sent out a message to employees announcing Sawyer would not be working for twenty-eight days. Addition-

---

[3] http://www.frontpageafricaonline.com/index.php/politic/2669-ebola-struck-closed-to-home-e-mail-explains-patrick-sawyer-s-thought

ally, the notification of his contact with Ebola was sent to Liberia's Ministry of Health.

Despite his direct contact with Ebola, Mr. Sawyer decided to travel internationally. On July 20th he flew to Nigeria, Africa's most populous country, to represent Liberia's Ministry of Finance at an ECOWAS (Economic Community of West African States) meeting. The plane landed in Lagos, Nigeria's capital city and home to a population of twenty-one million people.

Patrick Sawyer collapsed in the airport upon arrival. Mr. Abdulqudir, a Protocol Assistant for ECOWAS who had been sent to pick up Sawyer, helped him get to Lagos' First Consultant Hospital. At the hospital Sawyer was tested for HIV, AIDS and malaria. All came back negative. The staff became suspicious. When asked whether he had made contact with any person with the Ebola virus or had recently attended a funeral, Sawyer said no to both questions.

Because he was from Liberia, they insisted on drawing blood. Patrick Sawyer tested positive for Ebola. When told the diagnosis, Sawyer became angry and denied he had Ebola. He still thought he should attend the ECOWAS meeting. Dr. Ameyo Adadevoh vehemently insisted he not leave.

The disease progressed and on July 25, 2014, Patrick Sawyer died. He became the first American citizen to die of Ebola as well as the first person to die of Ebola in Nigeria during the current epidemic.

Sadly, others soon followed him. The ECOWAS protocol officer who met him at the airport died. On the very first night she worked at First Consultant, a pregnant nurse named Justina was infected with Ebola when Sawyer ripped out his IV and blood had dripped into her hands. A much loved and respected figure at First Consultant, Dr. Ameyo Adadevoh, came down with Ebola and died. She was praised after her death for playing a key role in curbing the spread of Ebola in Nigeria by preventing an irrational Sawyer from leaving the hospital.

These were just a few of the people whose lives were ripped apart when Patrick Sawyer imported Ebola to Nigeria.

Chapter 11:
Going Home

August 21, 2014 was a very wonderful and memorable day for us. After almost three weeks in isolation at Emory University Hospital, a gaunt but radiant Dr. Brantly walked before a crowded room of cameramen and women and their accompanying reporters. A bank of microphones had been set up for him at Emory Hospital and eager media personnel were there to record everything that was said. Standing with him was a large group of beaming staff members who had collectively worked to save his life. No one was beaming more than Amber. Her face was glowing as she stood near Kent, her hand in his. The big scare was completely over.

That morning, when a blood test confirmed no more Ebola was in Dr. Brantly's blood, an excited staff helped him leave the isolation room in which he had been housed since his arrival on August 2nd. He was able to hold Amber for the first time since he had dropped her and the children off at the airport in Monrovia on July 20th.

Dr. Bruce Ribner, director of Emory's Infectious Disease Unit, made a speech at the press conference. He discussed Dr. Brantly and Nancy's recovery process. He said that he and his staff were pleased they had had the chance to apply their training, care and experience to saving them and that Kent and Nancy's hope and faith had been an inspiration to everyone there.

As Amber stood nearby, Kent went to the microphones and gave a speech that was repeated around the world.

> Today is a miraculous day. I am thrilled to be alive, to be well and to be reunited with my family. As a medical missionary, I never imagined myself in this position. When my family and I moved to Liberia last October to begin a two-year term working with Samaritan's Purse, Ebola was not on the radar. We moved to Liberia because God called

us to serve the people of Liberia.

In March, when we got word that Ebola was in Guinea and had spread to Liberia, we began preparing for the worst. We didn't receive our first Ebola patient until June, but when she arrived, we were ready. During the course of June and July, the number of Ebola patients increased steadily, and our amazing crew at ELWA Hospital took care of each patient with great care and compassion. We also took every precaution to protect ourselves from this dreaded disease by following MSF and WHO guidelines for safety.

After taking Amber and our children to the airport to return to the States on Sunday morning, July 20, I poured myself into my work even more than before — transferring patients to our new, bigger isolation unit; training and orienting new staff; and working with our Human Resources officer to fill our staffing needs. Three days later, on Wednesday, July 23, I woke up feeling under the weather, and then my life took an unexpected turn as I was diagnosed with Ebola Virus Disease. As I lay in my bed in Liberia for the following nine days, getting sicker and weaker each day, I prayed that God would help me to be faithful even in my illness, and I prayed that in my life or in my death, He would be glorified.

I did not know then, but I have learned since, that there were thousands, maybe even millions of people around the world praying for me throughout that week, and even still today. And I have heard story after story of how this situation has impacted the lives of individuals around the globe — both among my friends and family, and also among complete strangers. I cannot thank you enough for your prayers and your support. But what I can tell you is that I serve a faithful God who answers prayers.

Through the care of the Samaritan's Purse and SIM missionary team in Liberia, the use of an experimental drug, and the expertise and resources of the healthcare team at Emory University Hospital, God saved my life—a direct answer to thousands and thousands of prayers.

I am incredibly thankful to all of those who were involved in my care, from the first day of my illness all the way up to today—the day of my release from Emory. If I tried to thank everyone, I would undoubtedly forget many. But I would be remiss if I did not say thank you to a few. I want to thank Samaritan's Purse, who has taken care of me and my family as though we were their own family. Thank you to the Samaritan's Purse and SIM Liberia community. You cared for me and ministered to me during the most difficult experience of my life, and you did so with the love and mercy of Jesus Christ.

Thank you to Emory University Hospital and especially to the medical staff in the isolation unit. You treated me with such expertise, yet with such tenderness and compassion. For the last three weeks you have been my friends and my family. And so many of you ministered to me not only physically, but also spiritually, which has been an important part of my recovery. I will never forget you and all that you have done for me.

And thank you to my family, my friends, my church family and to all who lifted me up in prayer, asking for my healing and recovery. Please do not stop praying for the people of Liberia and West Africa, and for a quick end to this Ebola epidemic.

My dear friend, Nancy Writebol, upon her release from the hospital, wanted me to share her gratitude for all the prayers on her behalf. As she walked out of her isolation room, all she could say was, "To God be the glory." Nancy and David are now spending some much needed time together.

Thank you for your support through this whole ordeal. My family and I will now be going away for a period of time to reconnect, decompress and continue to recover physically and emotionally. After I have recovered a little more and regained some of my strength, we will look forward to sharing more of our story; but for now, we need some time together after more than a month apart. We appreciate having the opportunity to spend some time in private before talking to some of you who have expressed an interest in hearing more of our journey. Thank you for granting us that.

Again, before we slip out, I want to express my deep and sincere gratitude to Samaritan's Purse, SIM, Emory and all of the people involved in my treatment and care. Above all, I am forever thankful to God for sparing my life and am glad for any attention my sickness has attracted to the plight of West Africa in the midst of this epidemic. Please continue to pray for Liberia and the people of West Africa, and encourage those in positions of leadership and influence to do everything possible to bring this Ebola outbreak to an end. Thank you.

In my wildest dreams I could never have believed that the media would be clamoring to hear about those first days in our little Ebola ward, but yet they were. I could never have imagined my friend Amber would be a part of an international media event, but yet she was. And in my darkest days of concern for his life I could not have envisioned Kent standing before this forest of cameras and thanking God for sparing his life, but yet he was doing just that.

While listening to the press conference I learned, along with the rest of the world, that Nancy had already been released, Ebola free, from Emory. I was thrilled by the news. David had his wife back. Jeremy and Brian had their mother again. Nancy could hug and kiss her grandchildren freely.

I felt I had my friends back

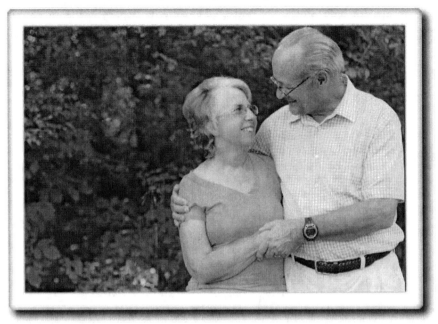

David and Nancy Writebol the day she was released from Emory University Hospital (Image - Bethany Fankhauser)

Chapter 12:
Dead Body Business

Liberians love what they call "dead body business." They say it ruefully amongst themselves all the time. "Dead body business" is anything pertaining to the preparation of the "dead body," (used in place of the word corpse), the wake and the funeral.

It is simply impossible to exaggerate how important the rituals surrounding death are in Liberia. Relatives and friends come from all around to comfort the bereaved when they hear news of a death. For hours, sometimes days, people sit quietly on chairs or mattresses on the floor while those closest to the deceased mourn.

Those following Christian traditions hold a wake the night before the funeral. Family members prepare the body for the wake by washing it and dressing it in his or her Sunday best. Large groups gather either in homes or churches and throughout the night they sing, give speeches and talk about how much the deceased will be missed. The casket is opened and all are allowed to express their grief freely. People may show their sorrow by kissing the body or throwing themselves across it.

Funerals are often elaborate. Churches are packed with mourners. The casket, prominently displayed, is covered with a specially-made family blanket and wreaths of artificial flowers. Often there are multiple musical specials and eulogies, followed by a full-length sermon. Mourners do not hold back. Often there is dramatic crying, especially from the women.

Muslims and those practicing African traditional religion also prepare their dead for burial with careful washing and dressing. All of this "body business" is very important in ensuring for the deceased a positive experience in the afterlife. Those not properly interned may become wandering spirits who will haunt the living. And in a country where "no one dies of natural causes," a funeral and all the "dead body business" that precedes it gives friends, relatives and even enemies of the dead the opportunity to prove to the deceased and to each other that they are not the ones who did the witching.

"Dead body business" changed completely when Ebola came to Liberia. In a country whose people know that to desecrate a body with an improper burial is to invite disaster, it was unbelievable that bodies were being placed in white bags, zipped up, and sent off to unmarked, mass graves. No church delegations sat with the bereaved. No wakes. No funerals. Not anything but the deep fear that those associated with the dead were now contaminated.

Things got even worse in August when corpses of Ebola's hastily-buried victims were seen floating in swamps. The rainy season's downpours had raised the already-high water table and lifted the white-bagged bodies out of their shallow graves. Horrified and disgusted, people feared their drinking water would be contaminated.

In addition to that, dogs were digging up the rotting corpses of Ebola victims, tearing open the body bags, and eating them. Dogs were also eating bodies lying on the street. Both the sight and the stench were horrifying.

In early August President Ellen Johnson-Sirleaf mandated cremation, virtually unheard of before the Ebola crisis. Rather than being buried, the white-bagged bodies of the dead were stacked on big funeral pyres and incinerated.

I came to deeply respect the men who picked up the bodies of Ebola victims. Day after day "body baggers," as they had come to be called, picked up the dead from homes, hospitals, or the street. Teams of four to eight men went to the death sites—the street, a house, a hospital—and picked up the corpses. Supplies were carried in the car in which they traveled. These included Tyvek® suits, buckets, sprayers with chlorine and body bags. Another vehicle traveled with them to transport the bodies.

Once at the site the body baggers donned their PPEs so the virus, which is most contagious at the point of death, would not infect them. The equipment included the footed and hooded suits, both latex and rubber gloves, facemasks, goggles, rubber boots, aprons and a second protective hood to be worn under the suit. I could only imagine how uncomfortable the men were in these outfits in the hot African sun.

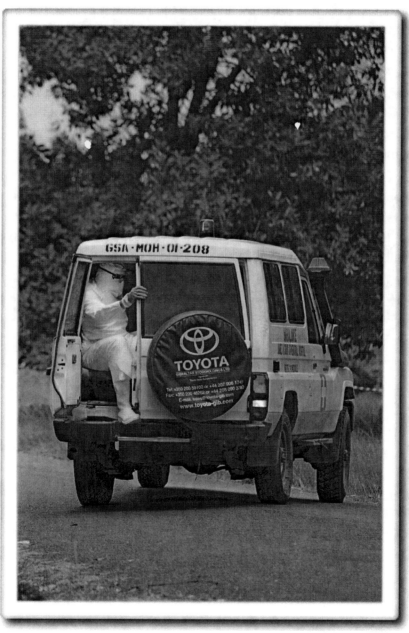

Liberian government ambulance (Image - Bethany Fankhauser)

If the body were at a home, a member of the team would spray the house with a chlorine mixture. This was done to protect team members and members of the household. The team opened up the body bag and placed it on the floor next to the body. They then sprayed the bag, the body and the entire area with chlorine water. After the body was lifted by the arms and legs and placed in the bag, the bag was zipped shut, sprayed one last time and taken to the vehicle outside that would take it away for cremation.

After the work with the body was finished, the body baggers were sprayed down with bleach water. Then they disrobed from their PPEs and carefully bagged what was trash. Their entire outfits, with the exception of the rubber boots and the rubber gloves, had to be burned or buried.

Perhaps nothing revealed more clearly the change in Liberia brought about by the Ebola crisis than the changed "dead body business." Because of fear, even the bodies of those who probably had not died of Ebola were being carried away by body baggers. Saying final farewells to loved ones had become potentially deadly.

Chapter 13:
Here We Go Again

In John-Mark and Sara's hometown of Voinjama, Lofa County, on July 29th at the Tellewonyan Memorial Hospital, several dozen Ebola patients were put in a room. They were awaiting transfer to the Ebola treatment center in Foya that was manned by Doctors Without Borders (MSF) and Samaritan's Purse personnel. For reasons no one knows, the infected people left their holding room and started wandering around the hospital, including the children's ward. Some were vomiting or excreting diarrhea.

A few of the Ebola patients wandered off the hospital's property and entered nearby homes. Within a short time the whole city was in a panic and for several hours it looked like a ghost town as citizens either escaped the city altogether or locked themselves inside their homes. All of the hospital's health workers fled in terror.

These were not the first healthcare workers to be terrified of Ebola and run. The domino effect had begun weeks before when both doctors and nurses were refusing to work in such hazardous conditions.[1]

A young nurse at Redemption Hospital in the Monrovian suburb of New Kru Town was the first healthcare worker in Monrovia to die of Ebola. In mid-June she unknowingly treated an infected patient. When she started feeling sick, Redemption's head surgeon, a Ugandan named Dr. Samuel Muhumuza Mutoro, treated her. He later died. St. Joseph's Catholic Hospital lost its director and several nurses after Patrick Sawyer's sister had been there.

---

[1] http://www.rappler.com/world/regions/africa/70583-ebola-hit-liberia-societal-breakdown

Official Ebola death tolls were mounting—both among healthcare workers and the general population. By the end of August more than one thousand four hundred people in the region had officially died of Ebola according to statistics, about seventy percent of those infected.[2] It would not be long before there were more deaths from this outbreak than from all previous outbreaks combined. The World Health Organization was admitting that the published numbers vastly underestimated the magnitude of the outbreak.

The World Health Organization (WHO) and Doctors Without Borders (MSF) were having trouble recruiting doctors from abroad in the numbers that were needed. In order to fight Ebola a doctor has to overcome fear for for his or her personal health on top of the many other hurdles of working in a country with which he or she is not familiar. Additionally the hours are very long and the heat of the tropics overwhelming in the already uncomfortable Tyvek® suits.

West Africa's Ebola outbreak was presenting very real and difficult-to-deal-with complications for health professionals and everyone else. Unlike previous outbreaks, this strain of Ebola initially lacked dramatic symptoms such as bleeding from the nose and eyes. Beginning symptoms mimicked malaria and cholera, causing frequent misdiagnoses. By the time the people knew what they were dealing with, others had been exposed and the patient's chance of survival had vastly decreased.

Unlike previous Ebola outbreaks that were limited to remote areas relatively easy to isolate, this outbreak spanned four overpopulated cities. In big cities like Monrovia, Ebola victims were difficult to find and isolate. Whole families were getting infected. In the interior of the country many patients were dying with Ebola because there were no open health facilities within traveling distance. There were unconfirmed reports of whole villages being wiped out.

Also unlike previous outbreaks where Ebola facilities were prepared for the number of patients known to need care, as soon as a facility was opened it was filled beyond capacity. Photos showed infected people sitting under trees waiting for beds to open up in the

---

2 http://www.sabreakingnews.co.za/2014/09/24/70-of-ebola-patients-have-died-who/

already overcrowded wards. Most beds became available by a death.

It is impossible to exaggerate how unprepared the medical community in West Africa was for this crisis. Prior to the Ebola outbreak Liberia had approximately fifty doctors in the entire country. Many clinics and hospitals had no electricity or running water. Often they had few medicines and their staff had limited access to diagnostic equipment. In some places medical professionals wore plastic grocery bags over their hands for want of gloves.

As clinics and hospitals closed, everything from malaria to childbirth became dangerous in a new way. With no available doctor to perform a cesarean section, a woman unable to deliver her baby dies, as does the baby inside her. With no one to help a diabetic patient, a treatable condition becomes deadly. The same is true for the patient with high blood pressure, burns or broken bones. Anything and everything could become a death sentence.

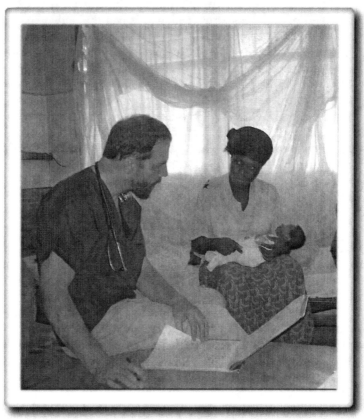

Dr. Sacra visits with patient at ELWA Hospital (Image used with permission)

After Dr. Brantly and Nancy Writebol had been struck down with Ebola, our friend, fifty-one year-old SIM missionary Dr. Rick Sacra, quickly returned to Liberia from the U.S. On Saturday, August 30, 2014, Rick posted a letter on his "iScripts" blog.

Dear Praying Friends,

If you followed the news over the last month, you have heard that ELWA hospital has been at the center of the Ebola crisis in Liberia. We are praising God for his mercy to our missionary colleagues, Dr. Kent Brantly and Nancy Writebol, who have been completely healed from the Ebola virus. They have been reunited with their families and are taking some time to rest and recover their strength.

The healthcare system in Liberia has had to go through a complete reboot after every single hospital in the city of Monrovia closed down to be decontaminated with bleach water as a result of Ebola cases landing in Emergency Rooms, outpatient clinics and medical wards. When I arrived on the 4th of August, ELWA hospital was in the middle of this process.

On August 6th, Dr. Brown, the medical director at ELWA hospital, opened the doors to Obstetrics patients. When the patients started arriving, they had often been to several other hospitals and traveled for hours seeking care. More than 35 cesarean sections were performed to save women and their babies in the first twenty days—sometimes two or three a day. This past Sunday when I was on call, several women presented for care in various stages of labor and three wound up requiring C-sections. One of them was a teenager with a full term pregnancy who had developed eclampsia, a combination of elevated blood pressure and seizures that would be detected in advance if she had been able to attend her regular pre-natal clinic. She was brought by her family, sprawled across the back seat of a taxi, unresponsive and still seizing occasionally. We had to give her a general anesthetic and perform an emergency cesarean. She is doing well now with her baby and will soon go home.

There are other medical emergencies that cannot be neglected much longer. Last week, I had a phone call from a friend to appeal for their neighbor, a 13-year-old girl who was very sick with severe abdominal pain. They had been to several hospitals but none was able to accept her. The family was desperate. Dr. Brown, who is a general surgeon, agreed to evaluate her even though the hospital was only open for obstetrics. Her exam indicated peritonitis, an infection in her abdomen, which would definitely require surgery. We waited all day Sunday for Dr. Brown who was busy caring for critically ill Ebola patients in the treatment center. Finally he came to see Lisa at around 8:30 p.m. after what had already been an exhausting day. It was clear that her surgery could not be put off, so we started operating at about 10 p.m. and ended after midnight. Dr. Brown found four separate holes in her intestine—perforations due to a typhoid fever infection. Each hole had to be repaired and then her abdomen had to be washed out. I spent the night on the pediatric ward monitoring her progress post-op, as she was quite ill with fever and difficulty breathing after the surgery. Today I am happy to report that Lisa is improving and slowly recovering. But she is just one of so many people in Liberia who are at risk because of the Ebola tsunami that swept through an already fragile healthcare system.

We are getting news now that a couple other smaller facilities in Monrovia are opening, allowing ELWA Hospital to open soon for additional services without being overwhelmed with a huge flood of patients. On Thursday, the 28th, we held a training session for all of our staff to review new triage procedures and infection control techniques to help protect us from unknowingly getting exposed to the Ebola virus. We hope to gradually increase our services over the next couple of weeks to include children and adults, but we must first make some changes to our building to allow us to triage everyone before they enter the hospital grounds to check for any signs of Ebola Virus Disease (EVD). A large shipment of personal protective gear arrived yesterday from our partner, Samaritan's Purse. This has been one of the key issues in reopening—ensuring that we have adequate protective equipment. So we are praising God for that!

Meanwhile, the number of people contracting Ebola continues to rise. WHO predicts the final numbers will be in the tens of thousands. The isolation and treatment wards on our property are packed and patients continue to come. While I am not involved in the units, Dr. Brown is passionate about ensuring they provide the best possible care so he is dividing his time between facilities. Thankfully, many people are surviving if they come when they first show symptoms. We rejoiced greatly that one of the ELWA nurses was released from the unit last week.

Please continue to pray! Here are a few requests:

1. That the international response to the Ebola epidemic will be vigorous! Right now, the systems put in place like ambulance transport and even the burial teams to dispose of bodies are overwhelmed.

2. Pray for ELWA's ministry at this time, that we would be able to make a difference for Christ in the lives of those who are sick.

3. Pray for the ELWA staff, for safety and protection from infection with Ebola.

4. Pray specifically for Dr. Brown and for Joe Wankollie, our SIM-ELWA Deputy Director who is running the whole show at this time. They are carrying a very heavy load.

In His Strength, Rick[3]

Under Rick's letter in the comments section my husband posted, "Rick, keep up the good work. We miss you and pray for you."

Only three days after Rick posted his letter on-line, as I was pulling weeds outside in the beautiful late-summer weather of Minnesota, my son John-Mark called me. I was totally unprepared for what he had to say. Dr. Sacra had just tested positive for Ebola.

No! No! This just can't be! I cried inside as a very shook-up John-Mark shared the few details he had. As well as being a friend, Rick represented the medical "face" of Liberia to me and now he had Ebola. This by simply working with maternity patients. I visualized Rick languishing in the Ebola ward in Liberia. I visualized Debbie becoming a widow. I visualized her three sons, my children's friends, losing their father. It was shattering.

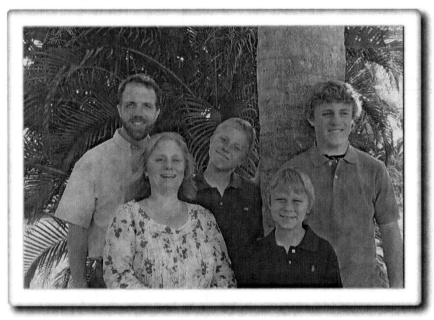

Rick, Debbie, Jared, Caleb and Max Sacra (Image used with permission)

We met Rick and Debbie when we were caught homeless in Liberia in 2002. We had been working with Liberian refugees in the Ivory Coast and making occasional teaching trips to the interior of

---

[3] http://iscripts.blogspot.com/2014/08/dear-prayingfriends-if-you-followed the.html

Liberia when the Ivory Coast's civil war broke out. Since it was now safer in Liberia than the Ivory Coast, for eight months we lived on the ELWA campus down the road from the Sacras.

Our friendship had been forged in the fire of shared adversity. As Monrovia started to fall apart again in 2003 and the tensions that preceded the rebel's last incursion into Liberia's capital city could be felt everywhere, we sought each other out for advice and encouragement. Even after the war ended and more missionary families came to Liberia, we remained close. Rick was always humble and approachable about medical problems and Debbie a wise and trustworthy listening ear. They were "Uncle Rick" and "Aunt Debbie" and their sons like cousins to my children.

Dr. Sacra's diagnosis with Ebola started an avalanche of news articles about him and the work he had been doing for many years in Liberia. Colleagues from the East Coast of the United States filled the airwaves and newspapers with praise for Rick's intelligence, kindness and dedication. I knew it was all true and felt humbled to have such a friend.

Debbie was amazing in the face of all of the media frenzy, especially considering she was dealing with her concern over Rick's condition. On September 4th, she stepped to the podium and with a perfect combination of poise and emotion, gave a speech we knew would make Rick proud.

I am overwhelmed and abundantly blessed by all the kind words that people have said about Rick since the news of his sickness was released. He will be somewhat embarrassed when he learns of it and he will say that all the glory goes to his Lord and Savior Jesus Christ. Thanks also to the Family Health Center of Worcester which has provided a professional home to Rick whenever we have lived in Central Massachusetts and UMass with whom he has partnered on the other side of the ocean, particularly in writing the HIV/AIDS guidelines for Liberia.

The Bible continues to be a source of comfort to me in the midst of this difficult time for our family. St Paul wrote "to me, to live is Christ, to die is gain – to depart and be with Christ is far better, but to remain in the flesh is more necessary on your account." We are indeed praying, that Rick will stay longer with us so that he can continue the good works that he has done in Liberia and also, caring for patients and teaching Family Practice residents in Worcester. But he would want you to know that he would not be afraid to pass into eternal life with the Lord, not because he has done good works, but because of the death of Christ on his behalf. The same love that Christ showed as he reached out to heal and comfort is the love that compels Rick: because Christ died for all, those who live no longer live for themselves but for Him.

Our mission, SIM (pronounced S-I-M), has been doing everything possible to care for Rick in his illness. They immediately sent an American colleague to Liberia to support the Ebola case management center director, Dr. Jerry Brown, in Rick's treatment and began the process of organizing his evacuation. My family is confident in the concern and attention of SIM and the ELWA family, as we have been for nearly 25 years. But our faith is in God's concern and attention most of all.

I would like to thank the media for their features on Rick this week. You have been kind and positive and allowed him to be an inspiration to our region. You respected my privacy when the news broke, and allowed others to speak for me when I might be too emotional to speak for myself. Rick and I have a close and loving marriage and his trips to Liberia are a part of our lives but that doesn't make them easy. When he left at the beginning of August, we understood there was a risk he could become sick with this deadly virus but I knew that he needed to go and be with the Liberian people who needed a hospital to be open. He was so concerned about the children who were going to die from malaria without hospitalization and the women who had no place to deliver their baby by cesarean section. He is not someone who can stand back when there is a need that he can take care of. His word to everyone who is watching these broadcasts is that the need in West Africa is desperate and there are resources that can be deployed to make sure that all healthcare workers have enough gloves and gowns and boots and thermometers to protect themselves from possible Ebola exposures and continue caring for those who need other medical care. Please find a practical way to meet the needs of Liberia and its neighbors in this time of fear and suffering. As Rick wrote to his medical colleagues, this epidemic is a wildfire about to rage out of control.[4]

To Mark's amusement, after Debbie's speech I sat in front of the computer and clapped. I couldn't help it. I was so very proud of my friend!

Details of his illness started to trickle out of Liberia. Rick had known it was a bad sign when he had started running a fever. He called Debbie and told her it was not good; he suspected Ebola. A

---

[4] http://www.bostonglobe.com/metro/2014/09/04/bgcom-sacrastatement/
Rhd6lfvaPC82lkcobyD6SN/story.html

blood test was done and they waited for the lab report to come in. When it did, it was positive. Rick moved from his house to the Ebola ward so Dr. Brown, along with the other staff, could care for him.

With no other surgeon in town, Rick had performed dozens of emergency C-sections. Many of the local hospital staff had been afraid to come to work after Dr. Brantly and Nancy Writebol's illnesses, so Rick acted as both surgeon and nurse much of the time. And while he protected himself with normal surgical garb, he had not worn PPE. Somehow he had been exposed to Ebola.

Happily, almost before it seemed like it could possibly be true, a plane had been arranged to transport Rick to the U.S. He arrived in Omaha, Nebraska on September 5th and was taken by ambulance to the Nebraska Medical Center.

The hospital staff gave Rick everything they could get their hands on that might possibly help him. They carefully balanced his electrolytes to keep his heart and other organs functioning as they should. Rick received a research drug called TKM-Ebola[5] for a week.[6] Dr. Brantly and Rick both knew that the blood given to Kent from Gartee may have been a factor in his survival, so Kent immediately flew out from North Carolina to Nebraska to donate a unit of his plasma.

Debbie kept her friends on Facebook informed about what was going on with Rick. We were encouraged as his health, after some rough days, began to noticeably improve. It was a happy day when Debbie announced that Rick had found Ben and Jerry's Cookie Dough ice cream to be, quite literally, just what the doctor ordered. He had been told he needed to eat 1200 calories each day and, lo and behold, he had done just that with ice cream.

We decided to pay Rick a visit in Omaha. Rick and Debbie's son Max was at the hospital and met us outside. Debbie had gone back to the East Coast to take care of some personal matters. We were taken to a small lounge. Outside of it at a desk sat a security guard, placed there to protect the hospital's special biocontainment unit—in

---

[5] http://www.tekmira.com/pipeline/tkm-ebola.php

[6] http://www.simusa.org/content/prayer-blog/page-13/4731/doctors_release_name _of_ research_drug_given_to_dr_sacra

other words, Rick.

Max made the video chat connection and, after a pause, Rick appeared. He was in bed and wearing a hospital gown, but to us he looked great. It was wonderful to hear his voice, see his smile and hear his laughter. For an hour and a half we talked of Liberia, Ebola strategy, Debbie and his health. It was bizarre to be so close to Rick—in the same building—and to be talking this way. As the conversation ebbed and flowed from the personal to the professional and back again, the video monitor was forgotten and it was a little taste of our Liberian home.

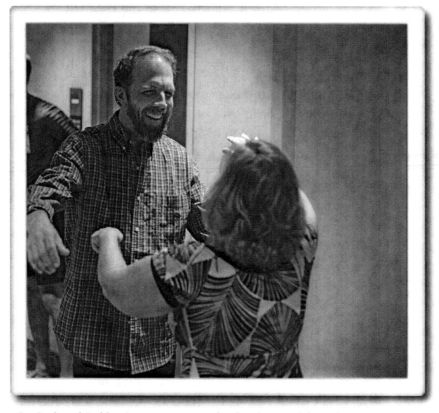

Dr. Rick and Debbie Sacra reuniting after his dismissal from the isolation unit (Image - Taylor Wilson, courtesy of Nebraska Medical Center)

A week later, on September 25th, a weak but Ebola-free Rick was dismissed from the Nebraska Medical Center. With Debbie at his side, he sat before a crowded room and praised God for His goodness to them. I was thrilled that God had, once again, spared the life of a friend. I was also thrilled that the sea of reporters recording his dismissal from the hospital would, as they had with Dr. Brantly and Nancy, broadcast to the world what Christlikeness and its accompanying trust in God looked like.

Chapter 14:
Ebola Orphans

In retrospect I should not be surprised that it was my daughter Melodie who introduced our family to fostering children. She was a very nurturing little girl—bringing back baby animals from the brink of death, placing babies on her back and carrying them around as if she were a Liberian mother, and generally looking forward to having children of her own from the time she was a little girl.

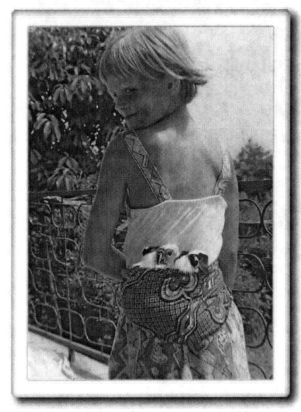

Melodie with pet guinea pigs - 1994

In 2005 Melodie flew to Liberia during her college summer break to fulfill an internship requirement. She was working with children at the Susie Guenter Orphanage near ELWA when she noticed a sick and pathetically skinny little girl. She had been abandoned on the streets of Monrovia the year before and brought by the police to the orphanage.

One day Melodie plopped herself down on our bed and, with great emotion, asked if we could bring this little one into our home for two weeks. She felt that would be enough time to figure out what medical issues the child was facing and begin to treat them. Mark agreed and, with the permission of the orphanage director, several days later we went to pick the little girl up.

Nothing could have prepared me for what I saw. Mary, whose age could not be verified, was thirty-six inches tall and weighed twenty-three pounds. Incongruous with her size, she had many adult teeth. A trip to ELWA's outpatient clinic revealed, among other things,

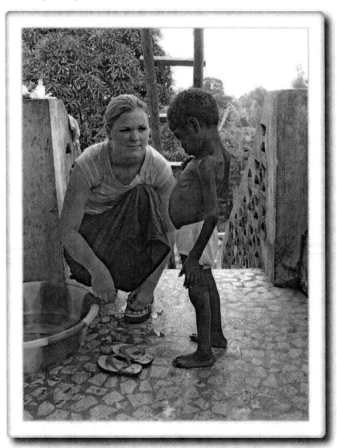

Mary with Melodie upon arrival at our home - 2005

chronic malaria, worms, scabies and an infection in her throat. Mary also had serious developmental issues.

She drooled constantly and was completely mute. But the most distressing thing of all was that Mary never smiled. I could only imagine what kind of abuse and neglect she had seen.

We started Mary on several medicines, which was no small challenge. She had no idea that this was for her own good and fought the combined efforts of Melodie and me with all of her strength.

The two weeks turned into eight months. We poured ourselves into this little girl and were privileged to watch a transformation unlike anything we'd seen before. By the time she went to an adoptive family in Canada, Mary had grown more than six inches and gained twenty pounds. Even more amazing than the physical growth was the emotional growth. She went from a fearful, withdrawn child to a giver and receiver of love.

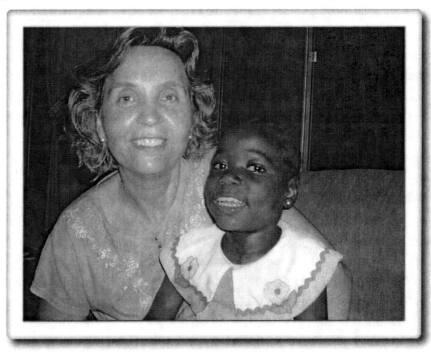

Nancy and Mary - 2006

My life was changed forever the moment Mary was placed in our care. She was the first of many children our family fostered and through them God opened our eyes and hearts to the heartbreaking world of orphans in Liberia.

A true orphan crisis is typically created when war or disease has ravaged a country. After Liberia's fourteen year civil war thousands of children were left as orphans. Hundreds of orphanages were opened to accommodate these children. Some single parents who were struggling to survive also left children at orphanages. Children were typically packed into substandard housing with a low caregiver to child ratio. In the years following the war these children were either adopted internationally, reunited with living relatives, or aged out of the orphanages.

Now, eleven years after the war, when Liberia's war orphan crisis was close to being resolved, Ebola created a new crisis. Tragically, losing parents to Ebola meant children became the victims of community-wide fear. For the twenty-one days after exposure, no one could tell the infected from the uninfected. Even grandparents or aunts, who in the past would have stepped in to help, were shunning the children whose parents died of Ebola. Rather than taking them into their homes and comforting them for their loss, out of fear for their own safety they were actively avoiding them.

To make matters even worse for the abandoned children, vendors did not want to serve them. These children were not welcome at the community wells. In some cases their houses were boarded up or household items destroyed because of Ebola contamination, making the children not only parentless, but homeless and completely desti- tute as well.

Such children were vulnerable in the extreme. After the war we heard horror stories of children who were tricked into sex traffick- ing, being lured in by false promises of food and shelter. Now, with Ebola killing parents and leaving children shunned, a similarly dan- gerous possibility was presenting itself. When the fear of contracting Ebola proved stronger than familial bonds, the children were left completely without protection from such predators.

I was so proud of my friend, Katie Meyler, whose face was showing up more and more in news articles. She had lived with us for two months a few years ago and we knew her well. Her burden for the vulnerable children of West Point, particularly the girls whom she feared would fall into prostitution, caused her to start the "More Than Me" foundation.[1]

Katie has the gift of seeing each person as just that—a person. When Ebola struck she was horrified. Especially so when West Point became a focal point of the struggle. She rightly recognized that Ebola terrorized children and unlike big, unwieldy organizations, "More Than Me" was able to flex to meet the epidemic's rapidly

---

[1] https://morethanme.org/about-us.html

changing and urgent needs.

Katie and her "More Than Me" foundation focused on locating and dealing with the sick in West Point. Katie mobilized an entire team of people who scoured the various districts to find the sick. If Ebola was suspected the person was taken to an Ebola ward. If the illness was likely something else, he or she was taken to a hospital. The response of the community was overwhelming gratitude.

As a result of her trips to isolation units, Katie found herself caring for several orphaned children. She, like others, found it extremely difficult to keep both the children and their caretakers safe as they waited and watched for Ebola's twenty-one day maximum incubation period to pass. But she did it and, by doing so, saved precious lives.

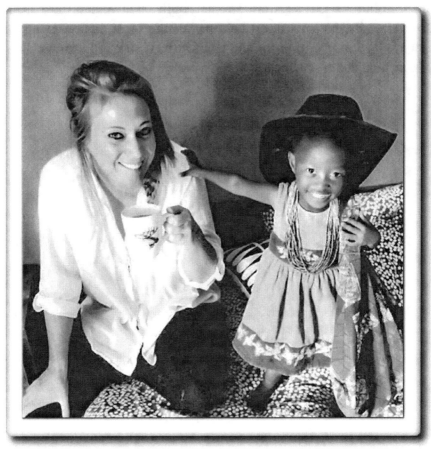

Katie Meyler with a Liberian child - 2014 (Image - More Than Me)

Of course Katie is not the only one helping these orphans. Specially trained Liberian nationals have begun partnering with local and international aid organizations to meet this unique need. Facilities are being opened to house these desperate children for as long as needed. For some, it is only the twenty-one day quarantine period after which they can be returned to a relative.

An increasing number of caregivers are Ebola survivors. These people are now immune and can provide the hands-on nurture and love infants and children so desperately need. In a beautiful yet heart-wrenching form of redemption, some are mothers who have lost their children to Ebola and are now eager to care for the needs of children who have lost their parents to Ebola.

This virus has created dilemmas that hurt to even think about and their solutions are far from simple. Sadly, one of the most heartbreaking dilemmas is that Ebola makes the most natural of all human affections—caring for and comforting a sick or hurting child—a potential death sentence.

Chapter 15:
Ebola Comes to Texas

We had been back from Liberia for a few months and my eighteen year-old son Jared had not been feeling quite right. His symptoms were not anything to be overly concerned about—just general malaise and a mild recurring fever. We decided to quit talking about it and have him seen by a doctor.

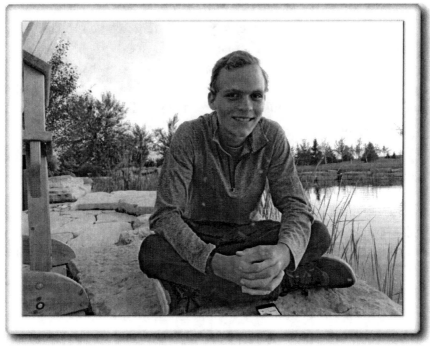

Jared Sheppard - 2014

Mark called a nearby clinic that seemed to have some experience with tropical diseases. He explained where we had been, when we had returned, and what we were hoping to accomplish by a visit to the clinic. Mark sensed fear rather than the curiosity a conversation like this would have generated in the past. When he finally had an appointment, the phone conversation ended with the nurse informing Mark that Jared would need to put on a facemask as soon as he entered the clinic.

Although nothing was ever found and Jared eventually recovered, we learned something very interesting through his illness. Ebola had put Liberia on the map. I should say that Thomas Duncan had had put Liberia on the map.

Thomas Eric Duncan was a Liberian man who lived on SKD Boulevard in Monrovia in a modest neighborhood of cement block houses with metal roofs. For two years he worked as a personal driver for FedEx's general manager in Monrovia. He decided to travel to Dallas, Texas, to visit his family.

Shortly before he left Liberia, Duncan's neighbor, Marthalene Williams, who was seven months pregnant, was in distress. Both Duncan and Marthalene's twelve year-old sister came to her aid. Together with family members, Duncan traveled with Marthalene to Monrovia's John F. Kennedy Hospital. After being turned away at both the maternity center and the Ebola ward, he helped carry Marthalene back into the house. The next day she died.[1]

Mr. Duncan traveled to the United States on SN Brussels Airlines on September 20th. Five days after arrival, on September 25th, Duncan went to the Texas Health Presbyterian Hospital in Dallas. He had a 103° fever, was vomiting and was suffering from abdominal pain. At the hospital he told the doctor that he had recently traveled from Africa. He was given an antibiotic. Three days later Thomas Duncan was brought back—this time by ambulance. He was desperately sick and suspicions were aroused. A test for Ebola was done. It came back positive.

The country went crazy. Even though there had been talk of what would happen should Ebola arrive in the United States, I do not think anyone could have predicted the tsunami of fear the first case would bring. While there had been a lot of press about Ebola in the past months, those pictures had been taken in Africa. Now the media

---

[1] http://www.nytimes.com/2014/10/02/world/africa/ebola-victim-texas-thomas-eric- duncan.html

was filming men in protective suits in Dallas. It was people in the U.S. who were now being quarantined.

Everyone wanted to know the full story. Reporters in Liberia went to Duncan's Monrovia home and found that Ebola was rocking the neighborhood. Nine were already dead or dying, including Marthalene's parents and sister.

In his isolated hospital room in Dallas, everything possible was being done to save Mr. Duncan's life. On October 3rd, five days after his arrival, Thomas Duncan was given the experimental antiviral drug Brincidofovir. Dr. Brantly offered his blood, but it was not a match. October 4th Duncan began experiencing liver and kidney failure and was given dialysis. Sadly, on Wednesday October 8th, he died. Soon after his body was cremated.

Apparently the protocols set in place by the Texas Health Presbyterian Hospital for treating Ebola patients were not sufficient.[2] On the nursing staff that served Duncan was a young lady named Nina Pham, a twenty-six year-old Vietnamese-American. She had done much of the care for Duncan during the eleven days he spent at Texas Health Presbyterian. Several days after his death, Miss Pham became feverish. She tested positive for Ebola and was transported from Dallas to Bethesda, Maryland, where she was treated at The National Institute of Health Clinical Center. Another young nurse who had cared for Duncan, twenty-nine year-old Amber Vinson, also contracted Ebola. She was flown to Atlanta, Georgia, and treated at Emory University Hospital in the same unit that cared for Dr. Brantly and Nancy Writebol. By God's grace, both survived their illnesses.

Thomas Duncan's story showcased a serious problem with containment. Because it is anywhere from two to twenty-one days after exposure before the victims start to show symptoms, people can leave their home country and be anywhere else in the world before they suspect they are carrying Ebola. And while we never wanted to find ourselves in this place, it appeared the United States was in a position to do what West Africa had failed to do—recognize and contain Ebola immediately.

---

[2] http://inthesetimes.com/working/entry/17271/texas_nurses_say_they_lacked_ proper_ protocol_equipment_to_treat_ebola

Chapter 16:
Abandoned to God

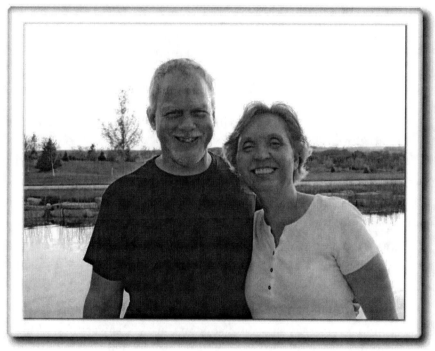

Mark and Nancy Sheppard - 2014

When Mark and I first announced we were going to Africa as missionaries, we were very young—twenty-five and twenty-two respectively. Most of our friends and some of our relatives did not know what to make of it. I suspect some did not believe we really meant it.

However, Mark and I each had a grandmother who did believe we meant it. And both of them were very concerned. Our grandmothers realized, much more than we did at the time, that the commitment we were making would come at great personal cost. Both were concerned that by obeying God's call on our lives, we would be saying goodbye to the good life they lovingly envisioned for us and saying hello to serious hardship.

They were right. After our first wonderful three-year term in Liberia, the civil war started. This thrust us into work among the Liberian refugees in the Ivory Coast, which was more challenging than anything I could have previously imagined. I had no idea that God *could*, much less that He *would*, ask something so difficult of me. I deeply resented the price it was costing me to follow Christ—how much I was being asked to lose.

I stumbled upon Matthew 10:37-39 and understood I had a choice. I could believe it was true or I could quit.

> He who loves father or mother more than Me is not worthy of Me. And he who loves son or daughter more than Me is not worthy of Me. And he who does not take his cross and follow after Me is not worthy of Me. He who finds his life will lose it, and he who loses his life for My sake will find it.

Because there had been so much that was truly agreeable during our first term in missionary service, it had not felt like a cross at all. In fact, I was under the impression I could "leave all" and still be having a good time.

Now I realized it was indeed a cross I was being asked to to pick up. But what did it even mean to do that? And what did it mean to "lose my life"?

I discovered the answer in Jesus' example in Philippians 2:1-10.

> Therefore if there is any consolation in Christ, if any comfort of love, if any fellowship of the Spirit, if any affection and mercy, fulfill my joy by being like-minded, having the same love, being of one accord, of one mind. Let nothing be done through selfish ambition or conceit, but in lowliness of mind let each esteem others better than himself. Let each of you look out not only for his own interests, but also for the interests of others. Let this mind be in you which was also in Christ Jesus, who, being in the form of God, did not consider it robbery to be equal with God, but made Himself of no reputation, taking the form of a bondservant, and coming in the likeness of men. And being found in appearance as a man, He humbled Himself and became obedient to the point of death, even the death of the cross. Therefore God also has highly exalted Him and given Him the name which is above every name, that at the name of Jesus every knee should bow, of those in heaven, and of those on earth, and of those

under the earth.

When Christ surrendered to the will of His Father to become flesh, live and then die that truly humiliating death on the cross, He was "losing His life." He surrendered not because He wanted to suffer, but "for the joy that was set before Him" (Hebrews 12:2). That surrender was the example I was to follow.

Many years later, on that first night I worked with Dr. Brantly in the Ebola ward, as dusk settled over the mission property he walked onto the porch. On top of a stack of papers on his arm he carried a book. It was *Oswald Chambers—Abandoned to God: The Life Story of the Author of My Utmost for His Highest.* He told me he planned to read it if time allowed. When I mentioned that I would love to borrow the book when he was done, Dr. Brantly insisted I take it. He doubted he would have time to read it right away. And so, in the wee hours of the morning and by the light of a flashlight, as aprons and boots soaked in chlorinated water, I read the story of a man who had lived out his relationship with God in the nitty-gritty realities of his daily life.

Indeed Dr. Brantly did not have much time for reading. More and more patients came to the ward. One long, hot rainy day followed another long, hot rainy day only to be followed by the long, hot rainy nights. I saw Dr. Brantly, Dr. Fankhauser, Dr. Debbie and so many others place the wellbeing of the patients above their own interests. The beating rain created a curtain between the Ebola ward and the rest of the world and in that small world, for these moments in time, we were working together and involved in something much bigger than ourselves. There was an otherworldly beauty to it. I was seeing Philippians 2:1-10 lived out before my very eyes.

While fighting Ebola was a unique experience for our team, it was certainly not the first time Christians had deliberately placed themselves in harm's way when dealing with pestilence. In the year A.D. 250 a terrible disease hit the Roman world. For sixteen years, city after city was decimated with up to five thousand deaths a day. It got so bad that even wars were halted. No one knows for sure what the disease was. All anyone knows with certainty is that it was an equal opportunity killer. The commoners died from it, as did Roman Emperor Claudius Gothicus.

Today we know about the plague because Cyprian, the Bishop of Carthage, described it as follows:

> This trial, that now the bowels, relaxed into a constant flux, discharge the bodily strength; that a fire originated in the marrow ferments into wounds of the fauces; that the intestines are shaken with a continual vomiting; that the eyes are on fire with the injected blood; that in some cases the feet or some parts of the limbs are taken off by the contagion of diseased putrefaction; that from the weakness arising by the maiming and loss of the body, either the gait is enfeebled, or the hearing is obstructed, or the sight darkened;—is profitable as a proof of faith.[1]

What was remarkable at the time was the reaction of the Christians to the plague. Rather than abandoning the sick and dying, they embraced the opportunity to help them. Cyprian says,

> What a grandeur of spirit it is to struggle with all the powers of an unshaken mind against so many onsets of devastation and death! What sublimity, to stand erect amid the desolation of the human race, and not to lie prostrate with those who have no hope in God; but rather to rejoice, and to embrace the benefit of the occasion; that in thus bravely showing forth our faith, and by suffering endured, going forward to Christ by the narrow way that Christ trod, we may receive the reward of His life and faith according to His own judgment.[2]

Throughout the centuries missionaries and many other followers of Christ have continued in this tradition. They were compelled to stay when others fled. Many were compelled to deliberately walk toward the danger—to be useful where needed, no matter what the cost. These people have not done it for fame or glory. Historically, when something happened to propel such people to prominence they reacted by throwing the light off themselves and on to those they were trying to help.

In this Ebola crisis there are a multitude of heroes, a few sung and many others unsung. These people are from all around the world as well as from the affected countries themselves. They are doctors and nurses. They are the people who, in spite of the danger to themselves, test blood for the Ebola virus. They are the people who wash linens and cook food for the staff and patients. They are the ambu-

---

[1] http://www.ccel.org/ccel/schaff/anf05.iv.v.vii.html, accessed Dec. 15, 2014

[2] Ibid.

lance drivers who pick up the living and the "body baggers" who pick up the dead. They are those who give their resources to make any of these things possible.

Sometimes in the darkness and quiet of the night at the ward, as I hung rubber boots upside down on sticks in the yard while rain ran over my head and down my back, I wondered how in the world I had gotten to this place. But, even then, I knew the discomfort was a small price to pay to be part of a team who together were fighting this most deadly of enemies. As a team we had a chance, "in lowliness of mind," to esteem others better than ourselves. We had a chance to look after the interests of others. We had a chance to be, both individually and collectively, abandoned to God.

Epilogue

My love for Liberia has followed a pattern not dissimilar to married love. My first years were flush with the romance of a new opportunity. Next was the middle stage when the warm blush of new love was gone. I could see the ugly bits—both Liberia's and mine. God did a transforming work in my life and this has carried me into the "old age" of my love.

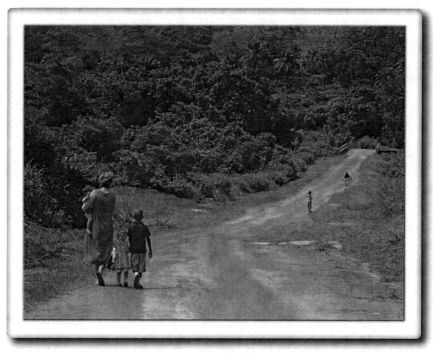

Nancy with Noah, Audrey and Jonah Sheppard in Voinjama, Liberia - 2014

I was enjoying its fruits when Ebola hit Liberia. For one month God gave me a chance to help in ELWA Hospital's Ebola ward and then He brought my family back to the States for Heidi's wedding. Because of a number of complicated realities, we do not know when we will return to our adopted African home.

I miss Liberia. But it is hard to explain what it is that I love and miss so much. I suppose it is not any one thing, but a combination of things. Maybe it is the way the ocean looks just when the fiery ball of the sun sinks below the sparkling horizon. Maybe it is the palpable relief I feel when the first rains come after a long and hot dry season.

Maybe I miss the crackle of an orange fire underneath a huge metal cooking pot. Maybe it is the anticipation that jumps up in me when I see a cloth-covered serving tray weighted with steaming bowls of rice and sauce. Perhaps it is the taste of hot pepper in almost anything and the pride exhibited by Liberians for being able to eat it without flinching. Or it could be that I miss drinking Coke from an icy glass bottle while sweat pours down my face.

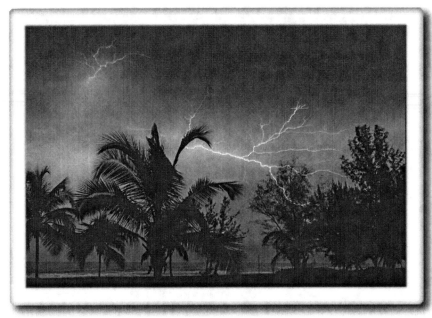

(Image - Bethany Fankhauser)

Maybe I miss the sound of a rooster crowing in the early morning darkness. Maybe it is the quick beep and rush of wind as a small motorcycle whizzes by. Perhaps it is the honking of a taxi's horn or hearing the voices of hundreds of people singing with abandon in a language both foreign and familiar.

Maybe it is the feel of rain water rushing over my sandaled feet as I hurry through the street. Maybe I miss ear-splitting thunder overhead as I lie snug in my bed. Perhaps it is the sight of clean clothes lying across the bushes, drying in the tropical sun. Maybe I miss the piles of cucumbers on rickety, wooden market tables looking at the same time both ordinary and exotic.

Maybe I miss drinking rich, chocolate coffee at the Royal Hotel with a friend and feeling pampered as we pretend we have no place else in the world to be. Maybe I miss hearing Mark's laughter as he sits in a circle of Liberian friends. Maybe I miss the sight of a mother, with a complete lack of self-consciousness, nursing her newborn. Or maybe it is the feeling of being a part of the sisterhood of women that fills me when I admire the baby.

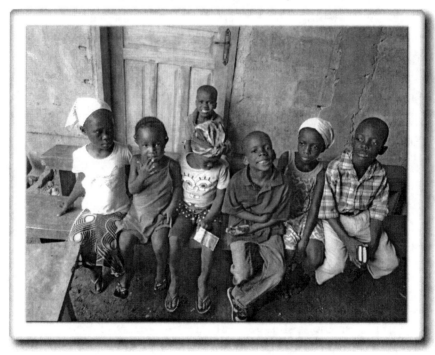

Jonah Sheppard (blue shirt) at Sunday school - 2014

Maybe I miss the unspoken community when dozens of people purposely wear matching clothes made of colorful African cloth. Maybe I miss seeing hundreds of uniformed children running around a schoolyard at recess. Maybe it is the children's voices ricocheting in the yard outside of a cement block church building while I, above the din, teach their mothers. Perhaps it is watching Jonah run around with those children who look so much like him and the sweet satisfaction of knowing that he will go home with me.

My family has lived and worked with Liberians since 1986. My heart beats to Liberia's unique rhythm. Its people have captured my imagination and their world is understandable to me. Sadly, as Mark and I contemplate the tragedy still unfolding before our eyes, we cannot help but conclude that so much of what makes Liberia unique—its culture, its history, its very personality—has created Ebola's perfect storm.

As I wait to return to Liberia I have had the opportunity to plug into the American life in a way I have not done for many years. That certainly has its advantages, not the least of which is traveling. Recently I was visiting my twin sister in Tennessee. Her pastor, Wes Alford, asked if I would tell the adult Sunday School class about my experience in the Ebola ward. Of course I was happy to do so.

I shared with the class the horror of Ebola and the honor of being able to help, if only in a small way, the effort to confront it. Everyone listened intently, clearly interested in knowing what it was like to be in Liberia at the epicenter of what had become world news.

Later that morning, at the end of the church service, the congregation celebrated communion. As piano music played in the background, small crackers heaped on a silver plate were passed from person to person. The crackers represented the broken body of Christ. After that tiny cups of grape juice, secured in a specially-designed platter, were passed. The juice represented the shed blood of Jesus.

When communion was over and it was time for the service's closing prayer, the pastor stood at the front of the church before the congregation and said thoughtfully, "I keep thinking about Sunday School and what Nancy said. It's all about the blood. It's all about the blood."

I recalled the story to which he referred. One dark night in the Ebola ward I witnessed a tragic scene. There was a young lady, Rose, who, although fatally ill, still had enough strength to wander around the room. She had moved a white plastic chair and was sitting just a few feet from where Dr. Debbie and I were sitting—she on her side of the threshold and we on ours.

Wrapped around her wrists were strips of gauze, placed there to stem the flow of her thin blood from the small holes where the IV lines had been removed. As Rose sat, her dark arms slightly outstretched, great drops of blood oozed through the gauze and splashed to the freshly mopped floor. Bright red, Ebola-filled, liquid death. All I could think of was getting it cleaned up, but I, of course, could not go past that all-important threshold. I could not clean up the mess.

Before the church congregation that Sunday, Karen's pastor contrasted the Ebola-ridden blood that brings death to its victims with the blood of Christ that brings life. I have, since that day, often thought of his words. Jesus put Himself in harm's way when He left heaven and came to earth as the God-man. He knew ahead of time He would face a cross, yet the sinless One stepped over the threshold separating heaven from earth. He did it to clean up the mess I, as a sinner, had made.

That blood fell at the foot of a wooden cross more than two thousand years ago, but it still has power today. The Bible says in 1 John 1:7-9, "But if we walk in the light as He is in the light, we have fellowship with one another, and the blood of Jesus Christ His Son cleanses us from all sin. If we say that we have no sin, we deceive ourselves, and the truth is not in us. If we confess our sins, He is faithful and just to forgive us our sins and to cleanse us from all unrighteousness."

Yes, Pastor Wes, it really *is* all about the blood.

Words of Appreciation from
Nancy Sheppard

No project is ever the work of one person, but never has that been more true than in the case of *In Harm's Way*. Without the dedication of thousands of people to the fight against Ebola, there would be no story to tell. So, first and foremost, I salute my dear friends with whom I worked in the Ebola ward and everyone else, in multiple countries around the world, who has helped in the battle against this most formidable enemy. Thank you, one and all.

The words, "assisted by Karen J. Gruver," on the cover are not there just to be cute or to be kind. Yes, Karen is my twin and I do realize it is quite sweet for us to write a book together. That being said, if she had not been pushing me from behind and working tirelessly alongside me, there would be no book. So, thank you, Karen. You're the best wombmate ever!

My husband Mark and son John-Mark worked behind the scenes to check and double check facts and help with formatting. You made *In Harm's Way* possible. Thank you.

Bethany Fankhauser, the teenage daughter of Dr. John Fankhauser with whom I worked in the Ebola ward, allowed me to include her photos in *In Harm's Way*. The reader can, through her lens, be in the Ebola ward with the team. Thank you, Bethany. God has truly gifted you.

Emily Sheppard, my daughter-in-law, was amazing. She was a great help in weeding out what bogged the story down and cleaning up what was left. Thank you, dear Emily.

Eric Buller, a longtime missionary friend and a coworker in the Ebola ward, along with his wife and children, shared information, encouragement and friendship. Eric, thank you for being there for our family.

Emily Gruver, my niece, kept my son Jonah happy while I was working. You're amazing, sweetie. Thank you.

Hugh and Marty McCampbell opened up their home to Karen and me when we needed privacy so we could concentrate. Their enthusiasm for the project was encouraging, their snacks delicious and their coffee energizing. Thank you, Hugh and Marty, for everything you did for us.

A special thanks to all of those who have loved and supported my family both financially and in prayer during our many years of missionary work in West Africa. You are appreciated more than you can ever know.

Thank you everyone who encouraged me to write Liberia's story and to all who read the manuscript and gave suggestions.

Lastly and most importantly, thank you, God, for everything. "Now to Him who is able to do exceedingly abundantly above all that we ask or think, according to the power that works in us, to Him be glory in the church by Christ Jesus to all generations, forever and ever. Amen." Ephesians 3:20-21

Other Books by Nancy Sheppard

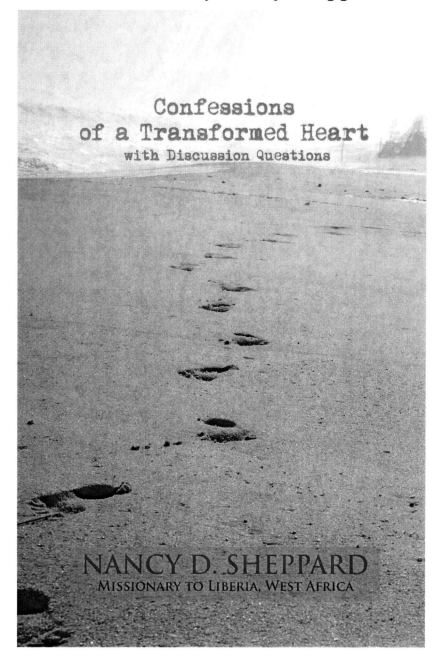

Nancy Sheppard writes of her experiences during Liberia's devastating civil war with the insight of one who witnessed the tragedy up close. Unable to return to their beloved Liberia after the young family's first term of missionary service, they chose to work among the refugees of the conflict in the neighboring country of the Ivory Coast. But this is not just a war story. This is the story of a woman transformed by the power of God in the midst of hardship.

> Contrary to popular assumption, meaningful work among the impoverished and war torn was not romantic, but was in fact quite the opposite. War refugees were simply people. People ripped from their homes, material goods and every vestige of normal life. Humanity at its rawest—all props gone. All of my props were gone, too. In place of the chipper, Proverbs 31 wife I imagined myself to be was a miserable, depressed, nagging shadow.

Follow the riveting story and see the transformation as God in His jealous love teaches the author about genuine service, submission, freedom, sincere prayer, reverence and humility. Scenarios you can't imagine, yet spiritual lessons with which you can fully identify.

For more information about *Confessions of a Transformed Heart* in English or other languages or as an audio book see www.sheppards-books.com.;

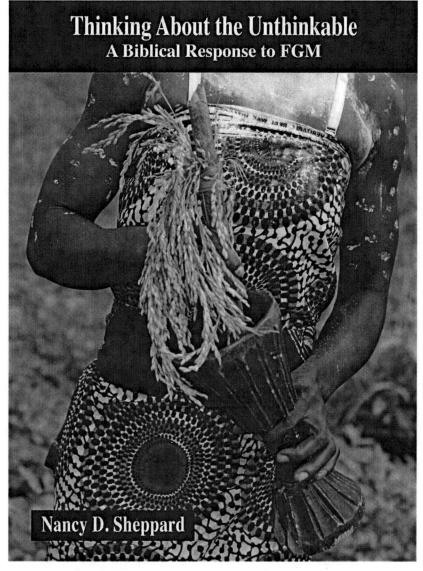

Thinking About the Unthinkable
A Biblical Response to FGM

Nancy D. Sheppard

Author Nancy Sheppard had never heard of female genital mutilation (FGM) until she arrived as a missionary in Liberia, West Africa, in 1986. In the decades since, because of her ongoing ministry among the affected women, she has studied the subject intensively. As a result, she has gained an understanding of the heart issues which lead to this painful and life-altering cultural practice.

Unlike the past, in this age of international travel, FGM now has the potential to touch anyone anywhere in the world. More and more often pastors, lay leaders and others in the West find themselves faced with questions and concerns about FGM—issues formerly reserved for those living in distant cultures.

Thinking About the Unthinkable: A Biblical Response to Female Genital Mutilation explains what FGM is, who is affected, the physical consequences and the reasons given by proponents for practicing female genital mutilation. The author uses scripture to identify the reasons this deeply embedded cultural practice is wrong. The last portion of the book focuses on how to counsel victims and potential perpetrators. Chapters include, "Instilling Biblical Hope After FGM," "Idols of the Heart and FGM" and "Fear and Female Genital Mutilation," etc. The author's goal is to prepare Christian counselors—professional and lay—to reach out with God's grace to those hurt by female genital mutilation.

For more information go to www.sheppards-books.com.

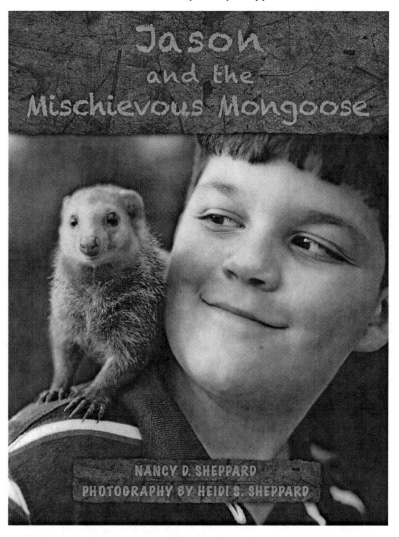

When nine year-old Jason Steward becomes the owner of a baby mongoose, he is sure that he can take care of him and keep him out of trouble. How hard could it be? But Pepper is as full of life and spice as Liberian hot pepper and Jason soon finds himself in a dilemma only God, though prayer, can solve. But where is God when Jason prays?

Written by missionary author Nancy Sheppard, Jason and the Mischievous Mongoose is a charming tale straight out of the jungles of Liberia, West Africa. Beautiful photography brings to life this missionary story that will delight readers of all ages.

133

For more information for this book in English or Spanish, go to www.sheppards-books.com.

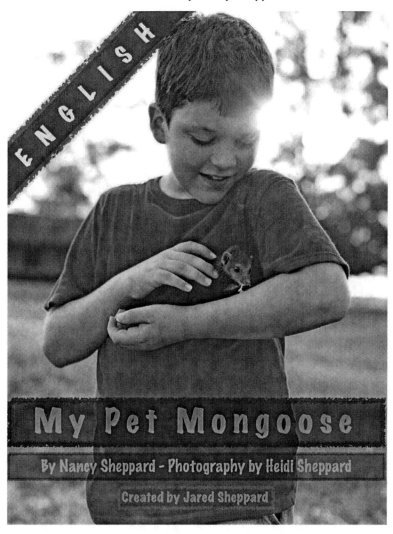

ENGLISH

My Pet Mongoose

By Nancy Sheppard - Photography by Heidi Sheppard

Created by Jared Sheppard

My Pet Mongoose is a colorful 4-in-1 beginning reader series the whole family can enjoy. Through brilliant photos shot in Liberia, West Africa, children are introduced to Jake, his American family, his Liberian friends and his mongoose Max. This charming introduction to the beauty of Africa includes the following four stories - "My Pet Mongoose," "My Best Friend," "The Color I Like Most" and "Who Loves Me."

For more information about *My Pet Mongoose* in English and other languages, go to www.sheppards-books.com

135